T5-CBB-006

Endoscopic Diagnosis in Gastroenterology

Endoscopic Diagnosis in Gastroenterology

Edited by

TATSUZO KASUGAI, M.D.

IGAKU-SHOIN   Tokyo · New York

Published and distributed by
IGAKU-SHOIN Ltd.,
    5-24-3 Hongo, Bunkyo-ku, Tokyo
IGAKU-SHOIN Medical Publishers, Inc.,
    1140 Avenue of the Americas, New York, N.Y. 10036

Library of Congress Cataloging in Publication Data

Main entry under title:

Endoscopic diagnosis in gastroenterology.

    Includes bibliographical references and index.
    1. Gastroscope and gastroscopy. 2. Stomach—Diseases
—Diagnosis. I. Kasugai, Tatsuzō. [DNLM: 1. Gastrointes-
tinal diseases—Diagnosis. 2. Endoscopy. WI 141 E54]
RC804.G3E53 1982   616.3'0754   82-9247
ISBN 0-89640-074-3   AACR2

© First edition 1982 by IGAKU-SHOIN Ltd., Tokyo. All rights reserved. No part of
this book may be translated or reproduced in any form by print, photoprint, microfilm
or any other means without written permission from the publisher.

Printed and bound in Japan

Foreword

In the preface to the first edition of Rudolf Schindler's classic book on Gastroscopy, published in 1937, Walter Palmer began: "The advance of science depends in large measure upon the development of objective methods... the two greatest contributions to the direct study of internal disease have been the development of the roentgenologic and the endoscopic methods." In the preface to the second edition of Gastroscopy in 1950, Schindler noted with satisfaction the general acceptance of the gastroscopic method and its rapid progress within the short span of a decade. The extraordinary technical developments in fiberoptic endoscopy since then surpass even the most extravagant expectations of its early supporters. I can recall my own collaboration with Dr. Schindler at the University of Chicago during the latter 1930's and our rather limited efforts to develop a gastroscopic photographic system. Technical progress in fiberoptics, bending capability, wide angle viewing, channel size and biopsy capacity now permit the relatively comfortable and revealing examination of not only the esophagus, stomach, and proximal duodenum, but also the colon, terminal ileum, and the bile ducts and pancreatic duct; areas of accessibility hardly anticipated in those earlier years. Endoscopy not only has advanced diagnostic approaches to gastro-intestinal disease but it also has enlarged our understanding of disease processes. It has provided much needed objectivity to therapeutic trials in peptic ulcer; and it has en-couraged the development of ingenious therapeutic approaches; techniques such as laser photocoagulation of bleeding gastric ulcer, the removal of stones from the common bile duct, and the removal of polyps from the colon; remarkable accomplish-ments in themselves. Endoscopy now facilitates the earlier diagnosis of colonic carcinoma and the identification of patients with inflammatory bowel disease at increased risk of colonic cancer. Endoscopy is one of the foundations of modern gastroenterology; an indispensable resource of the clinical gastroenterologist, an important adjunct for the gastrointestinal investigator, and an essential part of training for all students of Gastroenterology.

In the forefront of these impressive advances are the Japanese scientists and physicians, led by Dr. T. Kasugai and his six expert colleagues; each of whom has made important contributions to the progress of endoscopy. I can recall vividly my first visit to Dr. Kasugai's department at the Aichi Cancer Center, Nagoya, Japan in 1966; witnessing his remarkable endoscopy skills, and his comprehensive endoscopy program. From this contact there developed a long-term liaison with Dr. Kasugai and the Aichi Cancer Center and the University of Chicago, with well-trained young Japanese endo-scopists participating in the Chicago program in a collaboration which continues to the present time.

This book is a treasury of endoscopic information. Beginning with an introductory chapter on the central role of endoscopy in gastroenterology, the text deals with the esophagus, stomach, duodenum, endoscopic retrograde cholangiopancreatography, endoscopic sphincterotomy of the papilla of Vater, the small intestine and the colon in a concise and up to date form. The 141 case reports, 288 beautiful color plates and 150 radiographs constitute the central theme of the text and provide a highly informative and attractive documentation of diagnostic and clinical applications of gastrointestinal endoscopy.

This book will be of great value not only to students and physicians in training, but also to physicians and surgeons generally and, of course, to gastroenterologists. Spanning the 50 years from 1932 when the first semiflexible gastroscope was introduced by Schindler to 1982, the year of this publication, the book reflects the accomplishments of a modern master endoscopist, Dr. T. Kasugai, maintaining the tradition of excellence established by Rudolf Schindler, and is a fitting testimonial to his lifelong dedication to gastrointestinal endoscopy.

JOSEPH B. KIRSNER, M.D., Ph.D., M.A.C.P.

Louis Block Distinguished Service Professor of Medicine
The University of Chicago

Preface

At the present time morphological diagnosis of gastroenterological diseases is clinically made by comprehensive imaging, principally roentgenological examinations and endoscopy. Therefore, physicians who see patients with digestive diseases should thoroughly understand and master the procedures of digestive endoscopy as well as radiological diagnosis. This atlas of endoscopic diagnosis in gastroenterology was written to meet these needs.

After an outline of gastroenterological endoscopy, endoscopic techniques, procedures, indications, contraindications and complications involved in all of the segmental areas of the gastrointestinal tract and pancreaticobiliary system are described in considerable detail with selected references.

Approximately one hundred forty cases are presented by endoscopic color pictures combined with a coalescence of radiograms, macroscopic and microscopic pictures, each case accompanied by a brief history of the patient and laboratory data. The endoscopic pictures can be easily understood by the accompanying schemas. Descriptions of gastrointestinal diseases are also illustrated with a wide selection of endoscopic pictures together with various related pictures in radiology and pathology. This makes a written explanation simpler and clearer.

This book was written for postgraduate students, interns, residents and junior gastroenterologists, and it can also be used by endoscopists as a basic textbook of digestive endoscopy.

The authors of this book are all experts in the field of gastroenterology, and are internationally known as active and leading digestive endoscopists. Each contributed the chapter pertaining to his own gastroenterologic speciality. It is their hope that this book will become one of the basic textbooks in the field of digestive endoscopy, useful in the training, investigation and wider availability of endoscopic diagnosis and therapy for digestive diseases, and that it will benefit the correct diagnosis and better management of digestive diseases.

I would like to thank Joseph B. Kirsner, M.D., Ph.D., Louis Block Distinguished Service Professor of Medicine, the University of Chicago, for his highly appreciated foreword to our book, and H. Sugiura, M.D., Department of Internal Medicine, Aichi Cancer Center Hospital, for his help in preparing the microscopic pictures.

January, 1982   TATSUZO KASUGAI, M.D.

Contributors

MITSUO ENDO, M.D.
Professor, Department of Surgery, the Institute of Gastroenterology, Tokyo Women's Medical College, Tokyo

TATSUZO KASUGAI, M.D.
Vice Director, Aichi Cancer Center Hospital; Chairman, Department of Internal Medicine, Aichi Cancer Center Hospital, Nagoya

KEIICHI KAWAI, M.D.
Professor, Department of Preventive Medicine, Kyoto Prefectural University of Medicine, Kyoto

SEIBI KOBAYASHI, M.D.
Associate Chairman, Department of Internal Medicine, Aichi Cancer Center Hospital, Nagoya

MASATSUGU NAKAJIMA, M.D.
Assistant Professor, Department of Preventive Medicine, Kyoto Prefectural University of Medicine, Kyoto

KAZUEI OGOSHI, M.D.
Chief, Division of Internal Medicine, Cancer Center Niigata Hospital, Niigata

Contents

1

Endoscopic Diagnosis in Gastroenterology

TATSUZO KASUGAI, M.D.

Endoscopic examination is as important and indispensable as an X-ray examination in the clinical diagnosis of gastrointestinal diseases.

The original rigid endoscopes have been replaced by flexible fiberscopes which are in routine use for examination of the esophagus, stomach, small intestine and colon.

Fiberscopic examinations are performed much more easily and cause less discomfort and risk to the patient. They permit close inspection of the mucosa of the gastrointestinal tract with color photos and cinephotography if necessary. They are also widely used to obtain samples for cytology and biopsy specimens under direct vision.

Furthermore, visualization of the biliary and pancreatic duct systems by fiberscope — endoscopic retrograde cholangiopancreatography (ERCP) —, cytology, and biochemical analysis of directly collected pure pancreatic juice and bile, endoscopic surgery such as polypectomy and papillotomy — endoscopic sphincterotomy (EST) — have been performed.

Indications and Contraindications

The indications for gastrointestinal endoscopy include, in principle, all gastrointestinal diseases and will be discussed in detail under each procedure. Uncooperative patients and those with recent myocardial infarctions, severe pulmonary disease or infectious diseases, and cases in which insertion of the fiberscope is impossible are excluded.

Endoscopy is generally avoided in patients with known hepatitis B who give positive results when tested for HBsAg. If the examination is necessary, it should be performed as the last endoscopic case of the day, and the instruments used should be adequately disinfected using 2 percent glutaraldehyde solution or ethylene oxide gas.

Instruments

The forward-viewing fiberscopes are the most common instruments used for examination of the esophagus, stomach, small intestine and colon at present. However, there are specific gastroscopes and duodenoscopes which permit better visualization of the stomach and duodenum in certain patients.

Various models of gastrointestinal fiberscopes are available corresponding to respective organs, made by American Cystoscope Makers, Inc. (ACMI), Olympus Optical Co. (Olympus), Fuji Photo Optical Co. (Fujinon), Machida Endoscope Co. (Machida) and others are on the market.

Premedication and Post Endoscopy Care of Patients

The patient must be fasted after supper on the evening before the examination. About 30 minutes prior to the examination 1—2 ml of silicon solution is given by mouth to prevent foaming in the stomach and duodenum, also 5 mg of atropine sulphate is injected intramuscularly or subcutaneously to decrease secretion of saliva and gastric juice. Immediately before the start of the examination 0.2 to 0.4 mg of glucagon or an anticholinergic agent, e.g. 20 mg of Buscopan, is given intravenously, if necessary, to control peristalsis and spasm, and suppress secretions of the digestive tract.

Anesthesia of the throat is accomplished by having the patient swallow one spoonful of viscous Xylocaine.

When endoscopy is performed in outpatients, bed-rest is required for 2—3 hours after the examination until the effects of premedication and anesthesia have terminated.

REFERENCES

1) Endo, Y., Morii, T., Tamura, H., and Okuda, S.: Cytodiagnosis of pancreatic malignant tumors by aspiration, under direct vision, using a duodenal fiberscope. Gastroenterology 67: 944—951, 1974.
2) Hatfield, A.R.W., Whittaker, R., and Gibbs, D.D.: The collection of pancreatic fluid for cytodiagnosis using a duodenoscope. Gut 15:305—307, 1974.
3) Hirschowitz, B.I., Curtiss, L.I., Peters, C.W., and Pollard, H.M.: Demonstration of a new gastroscope the "Fiberscope". Gastroenterology 35:50—53, 1958.
4) Kasugai, T.: Evaluation of gastric lavage cytology under direct vision by the fibergastroscope employing Hanks' solution as washing solution. Acta Cytol. 12:345—351, 1968.
5) Kasugai, T.: Gastric biopsy under direct vision by the fibergastroscope. Gastrointest. Endosc. 15:33—39, 1968.
6) Kasugai, T., Kuno, N., Kobayashi, S., and Hattori, K.: Endoscopic pancreatocholangiography. I. The normal endoscopic pancreatocholangiogram. Gastroenterology 63:217—226, 1972.
7) Kasugai, T., Kuno, N., Kizu, M., Kobayashi, S., and Hattori, K.: Endoscopic pancreatocholangiography. II. The pathological endoscopic pancreatocholangiogram. Gastroenterology 63: 227—234, 1972.
8) Kasugai, T. and Kobayashi, S.: Evaluation of biopsy and cytology in the diagnosis of gastric cancer. Am. J. Gastroenterol. 62:199—203, 1974.
9) Kawai, K., Akasaka, Y., Murakami, K., Tada, M., Kohli, Y., and Nakajima, M.: Endoscopic sphincterotomy of the ampulla of Vater. Gastrointest. Endosc. 20:148—151, 1974.
10) McCune, W.S., Shorb, P.E., and Moscovitz, H.: Endoscopic cannulation of the ampulla of Vater: A preliminary report. Ann. Surg. 167:752—756, 1968.
11) Rebberecht, P., Cremer, M., Vandermeers, A., Vandermeers-Piret, M.-C., Cotton, P., DeNeef, P., and Christophe, J.: Pancreatic secretion of total protein and of three hydrolases collected in healthy subjects via duodenoscopic cannulations. Gastroenterology 69:374—379, 1975.
12) Schindler, R.: Gastroscopy: The Endoscopic Study of Gastric Pathology, 2nd edition. Hafner Pub. Co., New York, 1966.
13) Wolff, W.I. and Shinya, H.: Polypectomy via the fiberoptic colonoscope. N. Engl. J. Med. 288:329—332, 1973.

2

Endoscopy of the Esophagus

MITSUO ENDO, M.D.

With advances in the fiberoptic esophagoscope, esophagoscopy has been widely utilized by both internists and surgeons with significantly less pain for their patients because of the ease of its manipulation.

The present fiberoptic esophagoscope has some outstanding features. First, its operation is simplified. Using the push-button system of the control unit, aspiration, insufflation and irrigation can be controlled automatically. The head of the instrument can be bent in four directions: upward and downward, and to both sides. These movements make it possible to diminish blind spots in the esophagus and also make it easier to biopsy small lesions in the esophagus.

Instrument

Recently, the fiberoptic esophagoscope has been changed as follows: the bending angle of the head was increased up to 210 degrees with a radius of 1.0 cm. It can be easily bent while in the stomach even in a small remaining post-operative stomach (Fig. 2-1). The gastric cardia as well as the entire esophagus can be observed without blind spots. The esophagogastric junctional area can be examined with a frontal view, and a biopsy taken using the usual biopsy forceps at a position of maximal angulation (Fig. 2-2). This fiberscope can also be placed in the hernial sac of a hiatus hernia in the position of maximal angulation (Fig. 2-3). This examination is recommended for the evaluation of detailed alterations of the junctional area.

A TTL (through the lens) fully automatic exposure control mechanism has been built into the bright light source assembly (flash-type xenon light supply).

A small fiberscope (9 mm in diameter) has been recently devised. This instrument is very beneficial for use in screening examinations of the esophagus because of its painless manipulations.

Premedication

The patient should not be permitted to eat any food on the morning the esophagoscopy is to be performed. Fifteen minutes before the examination he should be given an intramuscular injection of 0.5 mg of atropine sulfate. Immediately prior to the examination the patient should gargle with 10 ml of 4 percent Xylocaine solution. In addition, Epirocaine jelly is used in some cases when it is needed. A sedative is also used for particularly nervous patients.

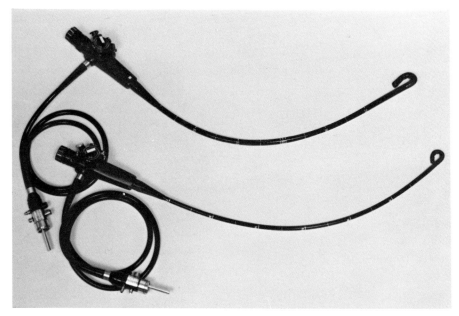

Fig. 2-1   Two esophagoscopes, Olympus EF-B3 (13 mm φ, upper) and Olympus EF-P3 (9 mm φ, lower). The tip of the scope can be bent to a maximum of 210 degrees.

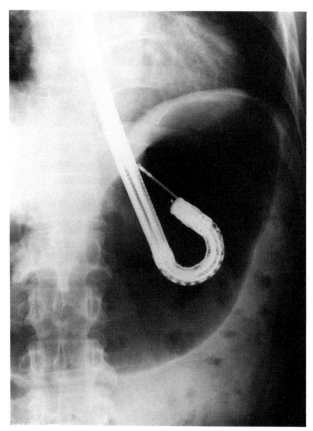

Fig. 2-2   After a "front-view" examination of the esophagogastric junctional area, a biopsy is taken with the tip of the scope maximally angulated.

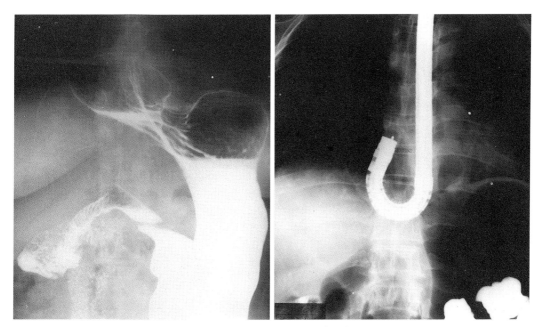

Fig. 2-3   An X-ray shows a paraesophageal hiatus hernia (left) and esophagoscopic observation of the hernial sac (right).

Indications and Contraindications

Fiberoptic esophagoscopy is performed on almost all patients complaining of esophageal symptoms during routine examination. It can be performed in a comfortable position for the patient. It may be performed safely on patients with bull necks or with kyphosis. To detect bleedings, it has also been done in cases with esophageal varices. Coughing episodes should be prevented during the examination.

Contraindications to fiberoptic esophagoscopy are severe heart disease, aneurysms of the aorta and acute corrosive esophagitis.

To increase the usefulness of fiberscopy, small fiberscopes have been utilized (Olympus EF-P3, GIF-P3, etc.). The small fiberscope is recommended in cases with severe strictures, for children and for patients with heart disease. Furthermore, the diagnosis of gastric lesions associated with esophageal cancers has been precisely revealed with its use.

Technique

The patient is usually required to lie on his back or left side. The control unit of the fiberscope is held with the left hand. The angle knob used to bend the distal end of the fiberscope to a desired angle is controlled with the left thumb. During the insertion of the fiberscope through the mouth and into the hypopharynx, the distal end may be kept slightly upward so as not to irritate the pharynx. When the fiberscope is inserted further into the hypopharynx, the insertion is facilitated if the patient is asked to swallow, while the instrument is being gently pushed forward with the tip touching the cricopharyngeal closure. In this way, the instrument can be smoothly inserted into the esophagus.

During insertion of the instrument from the pharynx to the esophagus, the following points must be taken into consideration: the insertion must be done under observation. If the tip of the instrument is kept turned upward and the larynx is thoroughly observed, the arytenoid cartilage may be irritated and painful coughing is caused while the instrument is being advanced through the hypopharynx. This can be prevented if the instrument is advanced to the mesopharynx with the angle knob being pressed forward to the "down" position with the thumb of the left hand.

After entering the esophagus, the fiberscope is advanced further with its field of view being constantly directed approximately toward the center of the lumen of the esophagus while feeding air little by little while occasionally suctioning and washing the lens surface. This is especially important for a patient with esophageal varices. The lower part of the esophagus has an axis deviation to the left but if the bending mechanism of the distal end of the fiberscope is properly manipulated, it can normally be inserted into the stomach under observation without any difficulty.

Therapeutic Esophagoscopy

Fiberoptic esophagoscopy has recently been used not only for the diagnosis of esophageal lesions, but also for the treatment of esophageal diseases.

Fiberoptic esophagoscopes as well as rigid esophagoscopes have been used to remove foreign bodies from the esophagus. Intragastric foreign bodies can also be removed in the same manner using a fiberoptic esophagoscope. A special forceps has been devised for use with the fiberscope (Fig. 2-4). Coins, fish bones, false teeth, apricot seeds and food masses can be removed using the fiberscope. Esophageal and gastric foreign bodies have been removed with fiberoptic esophagoscopy in more than 200 cases (Table 2-1). There have been no complications noted with removal of foreign bodies with the fiberscope. Local anesthesia is usually used to remove foreign bodies,

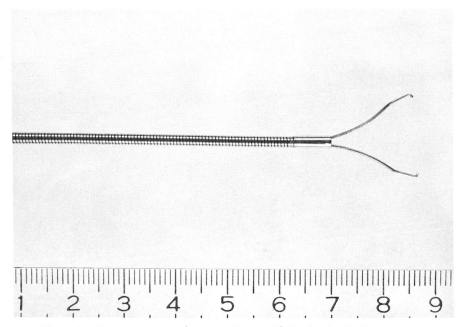

Fig. 2-4   Grasping forceps (interlocking teeth) for foreign body removal.

Table 2-1 Foreign bodies removed by fiberoptic esophagoscope (192 cases, 1979).

Food mass		154 (1)*
Meat	48	
Vegetable	32	
Fish	5	
Bean	7	
Sea food	6	
Miscellaneous	56 (1)	
Coins		16 (7)
Artificial teeth		5
Apricot seeds		3
Bone		1
Needle		1
Toy		3 (1)
Press-through-pack wrapping		1
Spoon		1
Tablets		5
Intraesophageal tube		1
Intestinal string		1 (1)
Total		192 (10)

* Figures in parentheses mean intragastric foreign bodies.

Table 2-2 Follow-up study of electrical incision (more than three months).

No stricture after first incision	53 (73 %)
Re-stricture	16 (22 %)
Satisfactory effect after second electrical incision	11
Required periodic bougienage even after a second electrical incision	4
Not effective after second incision	1
Relapse of cancer	4 (5%)

Clinically effective: 64/69 = 93 %

but general anesthesia is preferable in children and for patients with relatively large foreign bodies.

The removal of surgical suture material from anastomotic stoma is performed using a special "suture-cutting" forceps through the fiberscope.

A technique for polypectomy is used for the removal of esophageal tumors. A snare-loop forceps is used with esophageal lesions in the same manner as in polypectomy of gastric and colonic polyps. Submucosal tumors and polypoid hyperplasia of the epithelium less than 2.0 cm in diameter are resected electrically using the snare-loop forceps through the fiberoptic esophagoscope.

Enlargement of strictures is performed using a special electric knife through the fiberscope. High frequency electric current is used for this procedure. Electrical cutting has been used for postoperative strictures in cases of retrosternal, intrathoracic or intraabdominal esophagogastrostomy and intraabdominal esophagojejunostomy. The procedure was performed once in 73 percent of cases and more than once in 22 percent. It was successful in 93 percent (Table 2-2).

For urgent treatment of esophageal varices, embolization of variceal veins can be performed endoscopically. Ethanolamine oleate is injected into the varices through the fiberscope.

Elevated lesions in the esophagus are also treated by endoscopic polypectomy. Superficial submucosal tumors as well as pedunculated polyps can be resected by polypectomy.   After catching the tumor with a snare-loop forceps, high frequency current for electrocoagulation is used until the tumor is cut. Sessile tumors are also strangulated using a snare as though they had a stalk, and then removed in the same manner. At this time, without any complications, we have had the following experience: four leiomyomas, two hyperplastic polypoid lesions, one granular cell myoblastoma, and one lymphangioma. A tumor of up to 2.0 cm in diameter can be safely polypectomized.

REFERENCES

1) Demling, L., Ottenjann, R., and Elster, K.: Endoscopy and Biopsy of the Esophagus and Stomach, 2nd ed. W.B. Saunders, Philadelphia, 1982.
2) Endo, M., Kobayashi, S., Suzuki, H., Takemoto, T., and Nakayama, K.: Diagnosis of early esophageal cancer. Endoscopy 3: 61–66, 1971.
3) Endo, M.: Endoscopy of esophagus. In: Tsuneoka, K., Takemoto, T., and Fukuchi, S. (eds.) Fiberscopy of Gastric Diseases. pp. 215–223, Igaku-Shoin, Tokyo, 1973.
4) Endo, M., Kobayashi, S., and Nakayama, K.: Diagnosis and prediction of prognosis by endoscopy in superficial esophageal cancer. I to Cho (Stomach & Intestine) 11: 353–358, 1976. (in Japanese)
5) Endo, M., Yamada, A., Ide, H., Yoshida, M., Hayashi, T., and Nakayama, K.: Early cancer of the esophagus: Diagnosis and clinical evaluation. In: Murphy, G.P. (ed.) International Advances in Surgical Oncology, Vol. 3, pp. 49–71, Alan R. Liss, New York, 1980.
6) Japanese Society for Esophageal Diseases: Guidelines for the clinical and pathologic studies on carcinoma of the esophagus. Jpn. J. Surg. 6: 69–86, 1976.
7) Salmon, P.R.: Fibre-Optic Endoscopy. Pitman, London, 1974.
8) Savary, M., and Miller, G.: The Esophagus: Handbook and Atlas of Endoscopy. Gassmann, Solothurn, 1978.
9) Stadelman, O., Elster, K., and Ottenjann, R.: Esophagitis: Pathology and clinical findings. In: Maratka, Z., and Ottenjann, R. (eds.) Inflammation in Gut: Esophagitis, Duodenitis, Segmental Colitis. pp. 2–45, S. Karger, Basel, 1970.
10) Suzuki, H., Kobayashi, S., Endo, M., and Nakayama, K.: Diagnosis of early esophageal cancer. Surgery 71: 99–103, 1972.

Case 1 Normal esophageal mucosa

A 51-year-old male. *Chief complaint:* epigastric discomfort. He has complained of upper abdominal fullness and slight epigastric pain for two months. Gastroscopy revealed a small ulcer at the angulus of the stomach. Esophagoscopy was performed simultaneously, but no abnormal findings were observed.

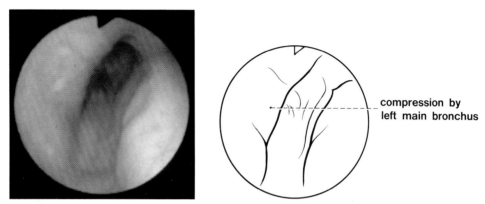

A. Normal mucosa of the mid-thoracic portion of the esophagus at the level of the bifurcation of the trachea. Compression by the left main bronchus is observed.

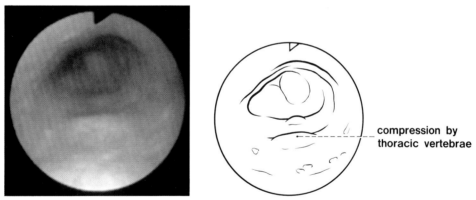

B. A more distal area of the mid-thoracic esophagus in which compression by the thoracic vertebrae is seen.

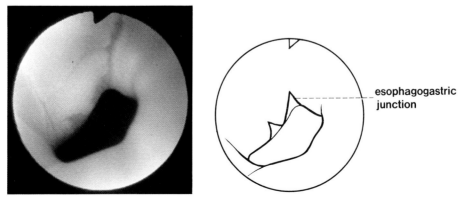

C. Lower esophagus. The esophagogastric junction is observed.

Case 2   Early esophageal cancer

A 55-year-old male. *Chief complaint:* slight esophageal pain with swallowing for two months. He had had a gastrectomy 16 years earlier after the diagnosis of a gastric ulcer. Laboratory data were normal.

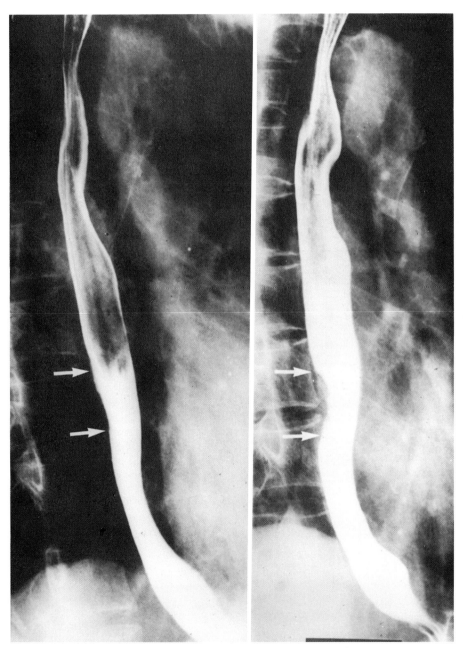

A. Right: X-ray examination reveals a superficial depressed lesion, 3 cm in diameter, in the lower esophagus. Stenosis is not seen. Left: Esophageal wall unevenness (arrows) is observed on the film taken during an examination six months earlier, but this finding was overlooked.

11

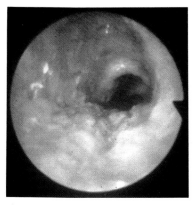
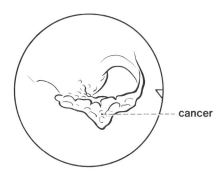

cancer

B. Esophagoscopy reveals a well-defined ulcerative lesion, the base of which shows marked irregularity.

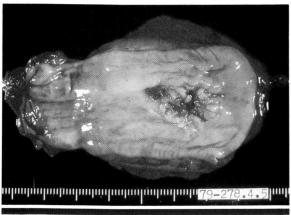

C. Resected specimen shows a well-defined, superficial ulcerative lesion, 2.5 x 2.2 cm in size.

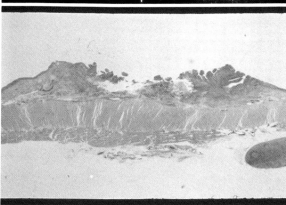

D. Histologic study demonstrates a well-differentiated squamous cell carcinoma in which invasion is limited to the submucosa. No lymph node metastases were demonstrated although slight lymphatic intraepithelial infiltration was observed. H.E., x 1.5

Case 3   **Early esophageal cancer**

A 57-year-old male. *Chief complaint:* mild epigastric pain for two weeks. Laboratory data were normal.

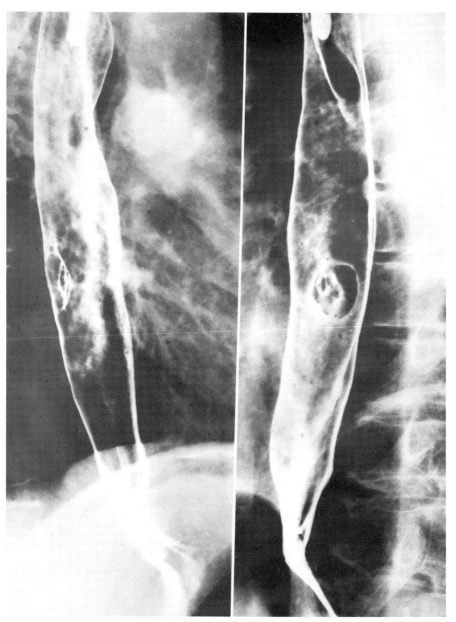

A. X-ray examination reveals a superficial elevated mass, 2.4 cm in diameter, in the mid-thoracic portion of the esophagus.

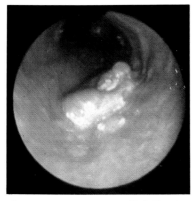
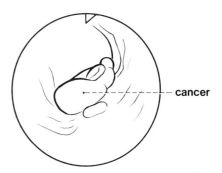

cancer

B. Esophagoscopy shows a well-defined, tumorous elevation on the posterior wall 32 cm from the incisors.

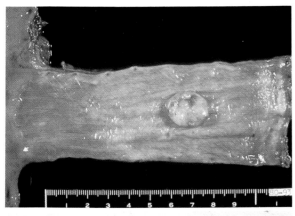

C. An elevated tumor, 2.8 x 1.7 x 0.5 cm in size, is seen in the surgically resected specimen.

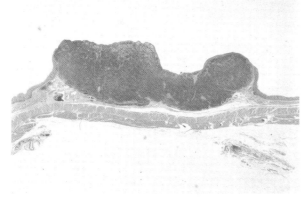

D. Low power histology demonstrates an undifferentiated carcinoma in which invasion is limited to the submucosa. Lymph vessels were extensively involved and metastases to the lower thoracic paraesophageal lymph nodes were also demonstrated. Hepatic metastases and pleural dissemination were not seen. H.E., x 1.5

Case 4   Early esophageal cancer: Lugol staining

A 68-year-old male. *Chief complaint:* asymptomatic. At a periodic health checkup, X-ray examination revealed an abnormal finding in the lower esophagus. Esophagoscopy was performed and biopsies demonstrated a squamous cell carcinoma. He was then referred to our hospital. Blood analysis and other biochemical investigations were normal.

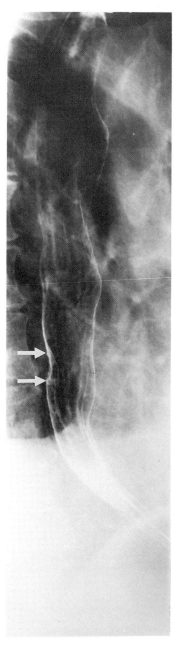

A. X-ray examination reveals unevenness and sclerosis of the wall in the lower portion of the esophagus (arrows).

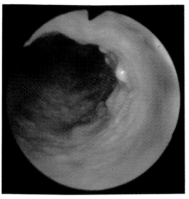
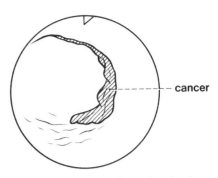

cancer

B. Esophagoscopy shows the erosive cancerous lesion on the esophageal wall, about one half of the entire circumference from the anterior to the right, with numerous fine granular lesions on its surface.

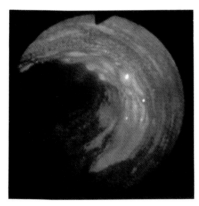
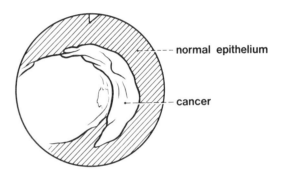

normal epithelium

cancer

C. Esophagoscopy performed after staining with 3 percent Lugol's solution. The normal esophageal mucosa stains black, but the mucosa of the cancerous region does not pick up the stain. The extent of the cancer is thus clearly defined.

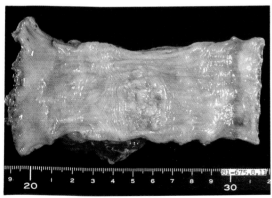
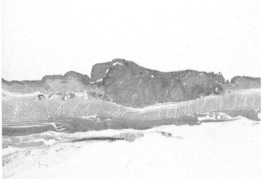

D. Resected specimen shows a superficial, almost clearly demarcated carcinoma, 2.7 x 4.0 cm in size, with numerous granular elevations.

E. Histologic study demonstrates a moderately differentiated squamous cell carcinoma in which invasion is limited to the submucosa. No lymph node metastases or invasion of lymph vessels were noted. H.E., x 1.5

Case 5   **Early esophageal cancer: toluidine blue staining**

A 61-year-old male. *Chief complaint:* asymptomatic. He had no symptoms referable
to the esophagus, but for the past three or four months he described easy fatigability,
even after mild exercise. Tachypnea was present. Upper GI series showed abnormal
findings in the esophagus. Blood analysis, biochemical study, pulmonary function
tests and ECG were normal.

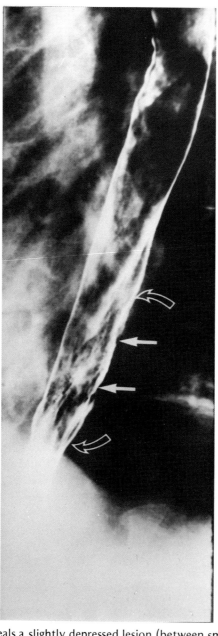

A. X-ray examination reveals a slightly depressed lesion (between small arrows) and roughness
of the esophageal mucosa (between large arrows).

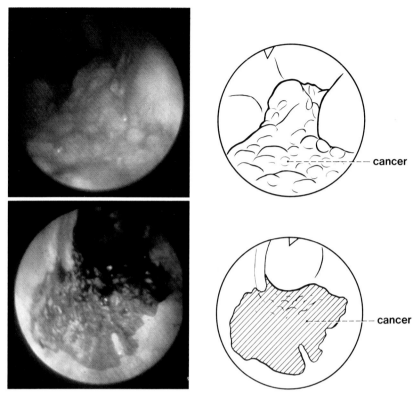

B. Esophagoscopic picture. Upper: Before administration of toluidine blue solution. A red, shallow, depressed, limited lesion appears with a deep ulcer. Its surface is rough with small granular changes. Lower: After administration of toluidine blue solution. The 2 percent toluidine blue solution is scattered on the esophageal mucosa through the biopsy channel of the scope and, one minute later, the mucosa is washed with water which is then aspirated from the channel together with the staining solution. The cancerous lesion stains blue and the border of the lesion can be clearly recognized.

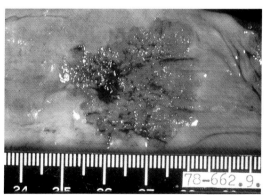

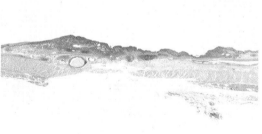

C. Resected specimen shows a superficial, depressed carcinoma, 3.2 x 3.4 cm in size, which has a rough surface and a moderately deep ulcer.

D. Histologic study demonstrates a moderately differentiated squamous cell carcinoma in which invasion is limited to the submucosa. Lymph node metastases were not noted — an early esophageal cancer. H.E., x 1.5

Case 6   **Esophageal cancer**

A 48-year-old male. *Chief complaint:* dysphagia for three months. Laboratory data were normal.

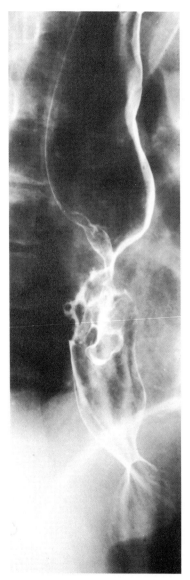

A. X-ray examination reveals a spiral-shaped filling defect, about 7 cm in size, in the mid-thoracic portion of the esophagus. Stenosis seems severe.

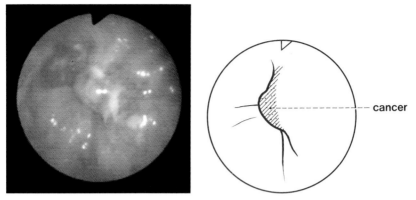

B. Esophagoscopy reveals a tumor 34 cm from the incisors involving the entire circumference of the esophagus. Significant stenosis is observed. A tumorous, proximal part of the carcinoma is seen on the right of the picture.

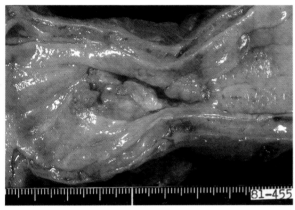

C. Resected specimen shows an ulcerated carcinoma, 4.7 cm in size, with marked infiltration of the esophageal adventitia.

Case 7   Cancer of the lower esophagus and gastric cardia

A 59-year-old male. *Chief complaint:* hematemesis. About one year earlier, initial bleeding occurred which subsided. One month before his visit to our hospital, hematemesis with melena occurred again. Nausea and abdominal pain were not observed. Laboratory data were normal.

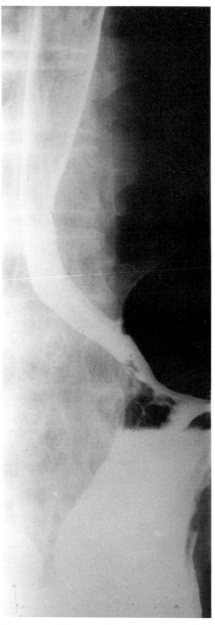

A. Unevenness of the wall and a filling defect are observed in the area from the lower esophagus to the gastric cardia. Stenosis is also present.

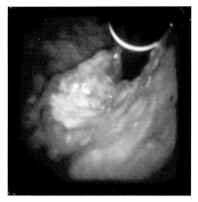 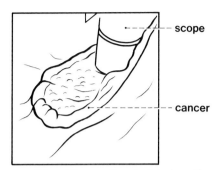

B. Esophagoscopy showing an ulcerated tumor with white coating just below the cardiac orifice. This picture was taken under retrograde observation.

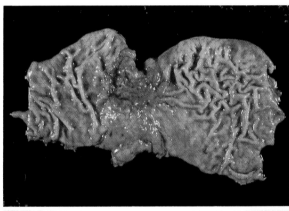

C. Resection of the cardia was performed. The resected specimen shows a clearly demarcated, ulcerated tumor, 5 x 4.5 cm in size.

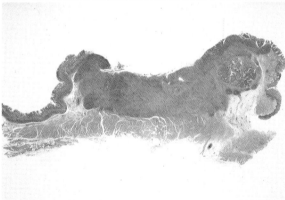

D. Histologic examination reveals a tubular adenocarcinoma. H.E., x 1.5

Case 8   **Intramural metastases of esophageal cancer**

A 73-year-old male. *Chief complaint:* esophageal pricking pain for about one month, usually when drinking liquor. He had no dysphagia or subjective symptoms. Blood analysis, hepatic and pulmonary function tests, and ECG were normal.

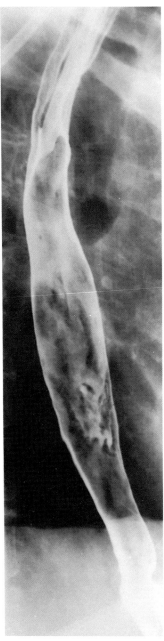

  A. X-ray examination reveals a superficial, depressed cancer in the lower portion of the esophagus. Small elevated or nodular lesions are seen in the oral side.

23

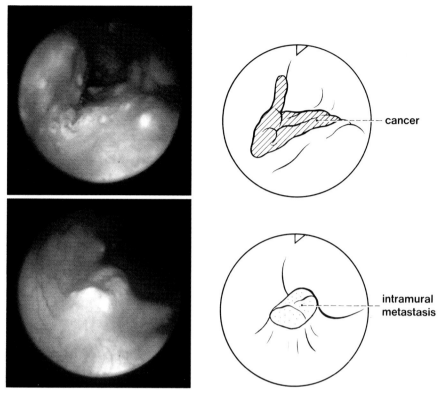

B. Esophagoscopy shows the main lesion of a superficial, depressed cancer (upper) and small nodular elevations on the oral side which were revealed to be intramural metastases (lower).

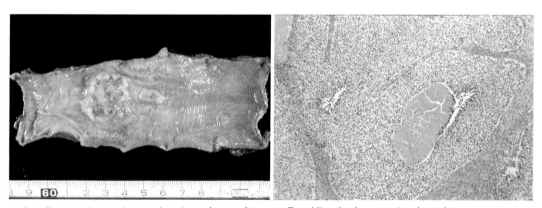

C. Resected specimen showing the main lesion of a superficial, depressed cancer, 3.0 x 3.5 cm in size, together with several intramural metastases of various size.

D. Histologic examination demonstrates a poorly differentiated, squamous cell carcinoma. The depth of the main lesion is limited to within the submucosa. H.E., x 40

Case 9   Esophageal cancer: radiation therapy

A 60-year-old male. *Chief complaints:* back pain and epigastric discomfort for about one month. There was no dysphagia, nausea or vomiting. Thirty-seven years earlier, he had had a gastrectomy after the diagnosis of a gastric ulcer. About seven years earlier he had also suffered pulmonary tuberculosis.

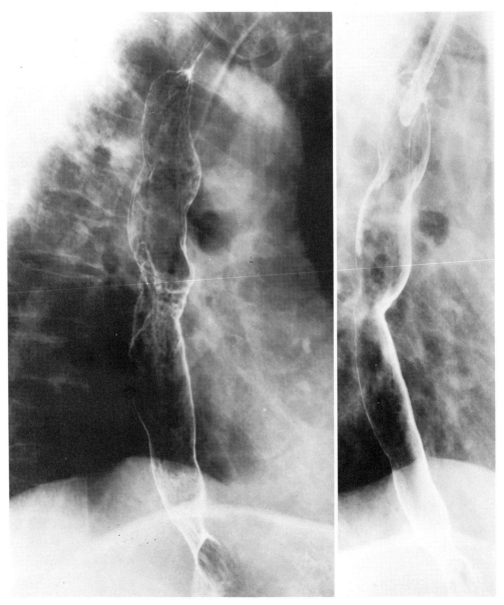

A. In the mid-thoracic portion of the esophagus, a serrated filling defect, about 6 cm in length, is seen on the right posterior wall (left, before radiation). A total dose of 6540 rads was administered to this patient. On the X-ray film taken after radiation therapy, the marginal elevations have already disappeared and only a slight, small depression is seen (right, 10 months after radiation).

25

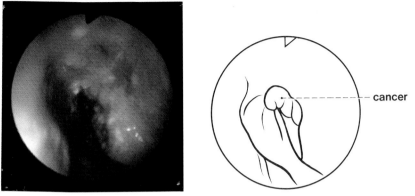

B. Esophagoscopy performed before radiation (Dec. 8, 1979). An ulcerated tumor is seen 33 cm from the incisors.

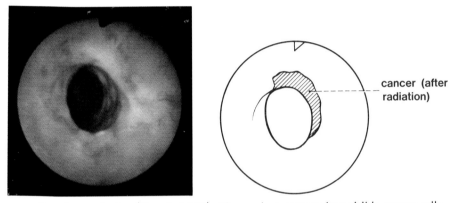

C. Ten months after radiation (Dec. 1, 1980). Biopsy demonstrated no visible cancer cells.

Case 10   Dysphagia lusoria

A 52-year-old female. *Chief complaint:* dysphagia. Because of dysphagia she had an X-ray examination performed. There was no heartburn or esophageal pain.

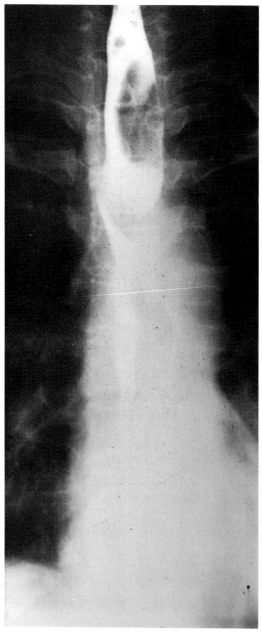

A. X-ray examination reveals filling defects in the upper thoracic esophagus. The margins of the filling defects are smooth. The mucosa appears normal.

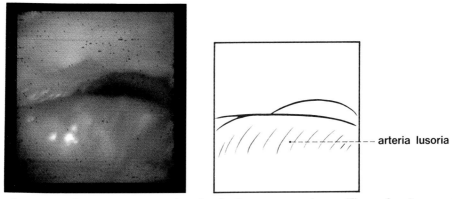

B. Esophagoscopy shows a tumorous elevation in the upper esophagus. The surface is normal and the scope could be passed into the distal esophagus beyond the elevation. The elevation runs transversely across the posterior wall of the esophagus. The diagnosis was compression by the lusoria arteria.

Case 11 **Foreign body**

A 82-year-old male. *Chief complaints:* dysphagia and esophageal pain. During dinner, dysphagia occurred abruptly as he had swallowed his false teeth with the meal. The next day, eight hours later, he visited our hospital.

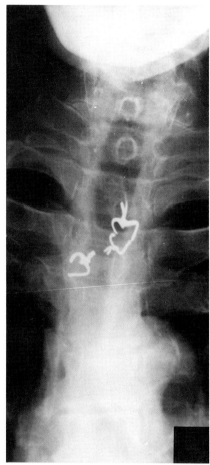

A. X-ray examination reveals the hooks of the false teeth in the upper esophagus.

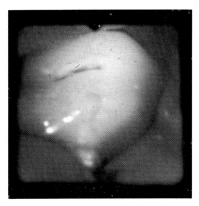 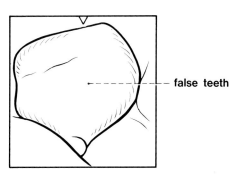

false teeth

B. Esophagoscopy showing a white tooth and metal hook. Following this observation, the false teeth were removed with a forceps through the biopsy channel of the fiberoptic esophago- scope under general anesthesia.

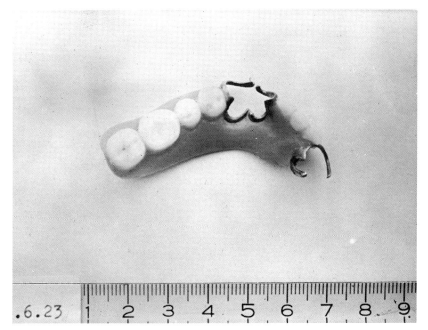

C. This picture shows the removed false teeth. After this procedure, he was able to eat food without any difficulty.

The flexible fiberoptic esophagoscope has been used recently for the removal of foreign bodies in the esophagus and stomach. Using a special forceps, foreign bodies can be removed with ease and safety. The role of the forceps is primary. A forceps with two arms is recommended for the removal of a solid mass and a basket-forceps for a soft or fragile food mass.

Case 12   Esophageal diverticula

A 63-year-old male. *Chief complaint:* longstanding foreign body sensation in the upper esophagus. He had intermittently complained of this mild irritation. No significant past or family history is noted.

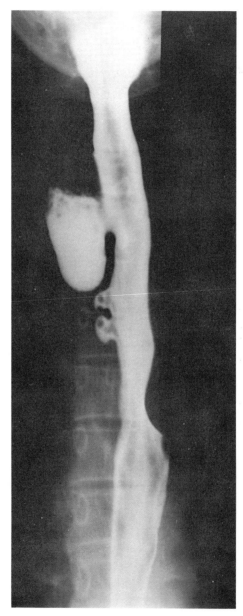

A. X-ray examination reveals a large diverticulum and two small diverticula on the right wall of the upper esophagus.

31

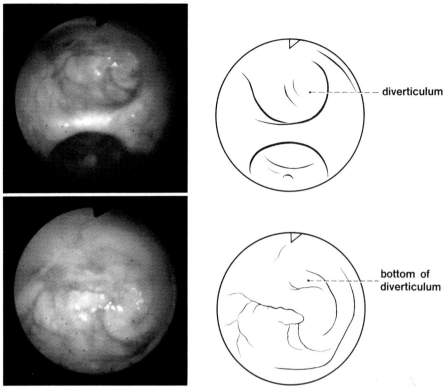

B. Esophagoscopic picture of the large diverticulum. The upper picture shows the esophageal lumen on the left and the diverticulum on the right. The lower one shows the base of the diverticulum. No inflammation is noted.

Case 13   Hiatus hernia

A 65-year-old male. *Chief complaint:* epigastric discomfort. There was no esophageal pain and his appetite was good. Laboratory data were normal.

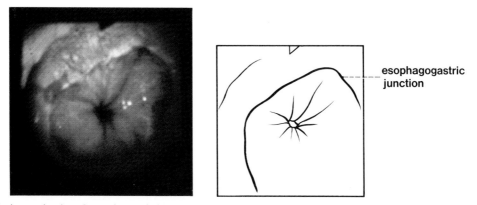

A.   Endoscopic view from the oral side showing a circumferential enlargement of the esophago-gastric junction. The gastric mucosa is seen through the enlarged cardiac orifice. Respiratory movement of the orifice is observed. This is considered to be a pinch-cock action.

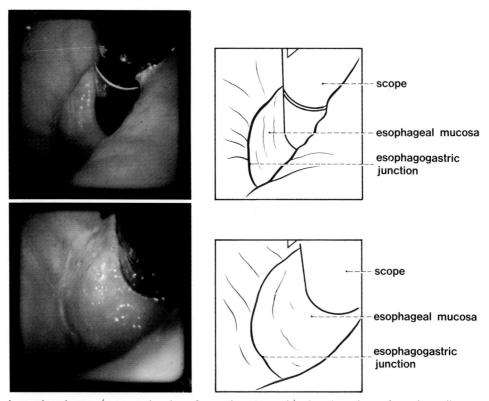

B.   Endoscopic picture (retrograde view from the stomach) showing the enlarged cardiac orifice. With the scope pulled close to the orifice, the mucosa of the lower esophagus is seen over the esophagogastric junction. In a close-up frontal view of the area of the esophagogastric junction, the esophageal mucosa appears to overlap the gastric mucosa.

Case 14   Esophageal ulcer

A 47-year-old male. *Chief complaints:* dysphagia and retrosternal pain. He had occasionally complained of difficulty on swallowing for twenty years and, after a diagnosis of esophageal ulcer, he had been treated medically. Surgical resection was performed due to recent unfavorable symptoms. He has no significant past or family history. Laboratory data were normal.

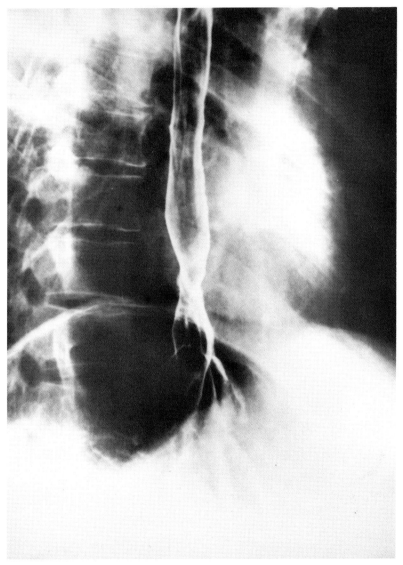

A. X-ray examination reveals a stricture of the lower esophagus with an irregular and sclerotic wall. The esophagogastric junction is pulled into the thoracic cavity. The esophageal mucosa proximal to the strictured segment appears to be slightly rough.

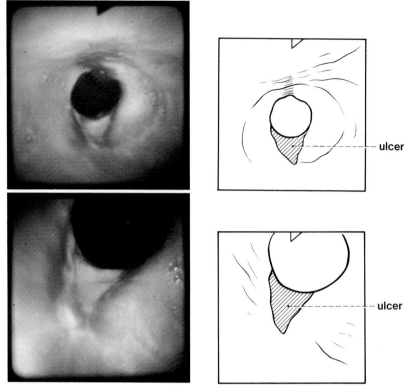

B. Esophagoscopy shows an ulcer covered with white coating on the posterior wall of the lower esophagus adjacent to the esophagogastric junction. Redness and roughness of the mucosa, findings similar to those in esophagitis, are observed at the ulcer margin, but a tumorous proliferation is not seen at its edge.

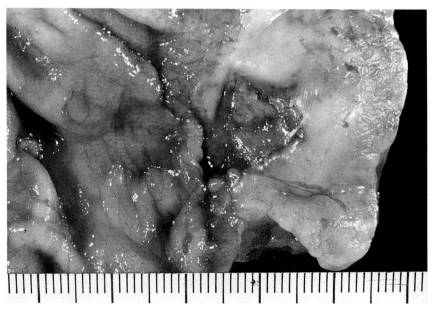

C. Resected specimen shows a well-defined, red ulcer, 1.4 x 1.4 cm in size, at the distal part of the lower esophagus.

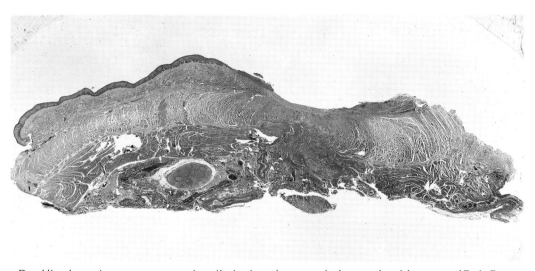

D. Histology demonstrates an ulcer limited to the muscularis propria with nonspecific inflammation. H.E., x 1.5

Case 15   Esophagitis

A 55-year-old male. *Chief complaint:* heartburn.

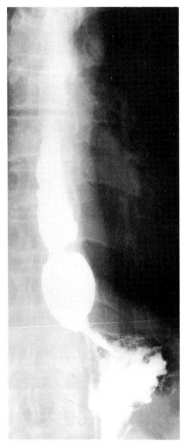

A. X-ray examination reveals a hernia pouch above the diaphragm compatible with the endoscopic finding.

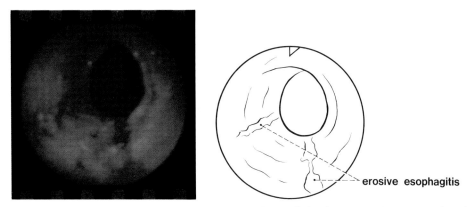

B. Esophagoscopy reveals patchy erythema and erosions of the lower esophagus associated with a hiatus hernia. The mucosa easily bled with instrumentation.

Case 16   Barrett esophagus and Barrett ulcer

A 59-year-old male. *Chief complaint:* retrosternal pain for two or three months. He had been complaining of heartburn for several years. His nutritional condition was good. There was no chest or epigastric pain. He had no dysphagia. Routine blood studies showed no anemia. Liver function tests and ECG were normal. The gastric acid level was within normal limits.

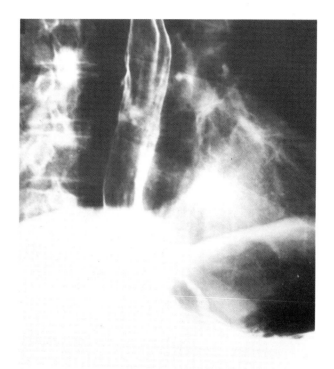

A. X-ray examination reveals a mild hiatus hernia without marked morphologic changes in the esophagus. Unevenness of the wall is noted in the mid-thoracic portion.

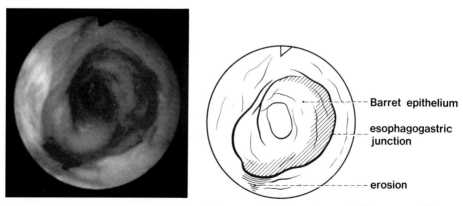

Barret epithelium

esophagogastric junction

erosion

B. Esophagoscopy shows a junctional area of the esophageal and gastric-like mucosa 25 cm from the incisors. The junctional border is clearly demarcated and esophagitis is observed on the oral side of the border. No stricture is seen.

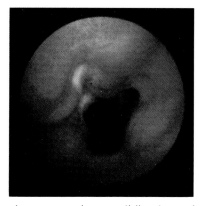 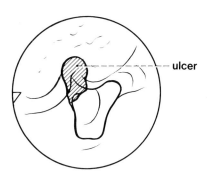

C. Esophagoscopy shows mildly deep ulcer, which looks like a gastric ulcer, on the right anterior wall 34 cm from the incisors. The ulcer base is covered with white coating. The epithelial mucosa surrounding the ulcer appears slightly rough with a red and poorly lucent surface.

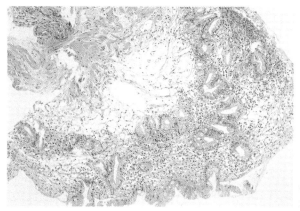

D. Biopsy demonstrates columnar epithelial cells which are apparently similar to the gland cells of the gastric cardia. H.E., x 50

In summary, this case is considered to be a Barrett esophagus associated with esophageal ulcer, a so-called Barrett ulcer. Although this patient had a mild hiatal hernia, the esophagus remained normal morphologically and columnar epithelialization limited only to the epithelial mucosa was observed. Medical treatment was instituted.

Case 17   Leiomyoma of the esophagus

A 28-year-old male. *Chief complaint:* asymptomatic. He was discovered at his company's annual checkup. Laboratory data were normal.

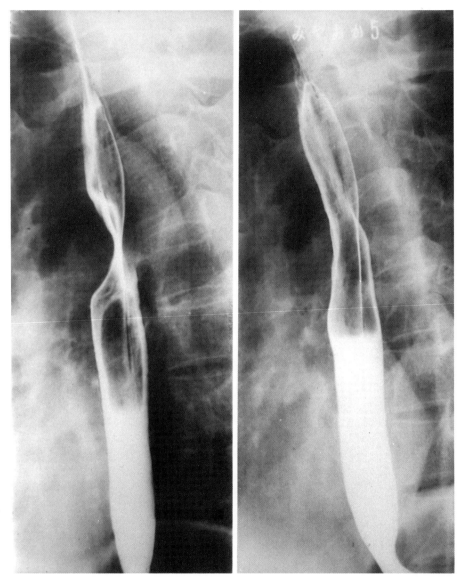

A.   Left: X-ray film before operation reveals a filling defect in the mid-thoracic portion of the esophagus, which suggests a submucosal tumor with a smooth surface. Right: Three weeks after operation. The tumor has entirely disappeared.

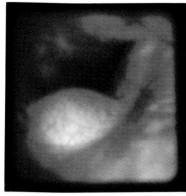
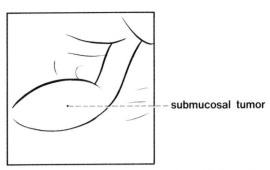

— submucosal tumor

B. Esophagoscopy shows a submucosal tumor with a smooth surface in the mid-thoracic esophagus.

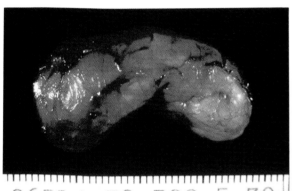

26514-72-320.5.30

C. Resected specimen shows a submucosal tumor, about 3 cm in size.

D. Histology demonstrates a leiomyoma of the esophagus. H.E., x 40

Case 18   Esophageal varices

A 45-year-old male. *Chief complaint:* abdominal fullness for about three months. He drinks about 360 ml of *sake* every day. He has no past history of gastrointestinal bleeding. No esophageal or abdominal pain is present.

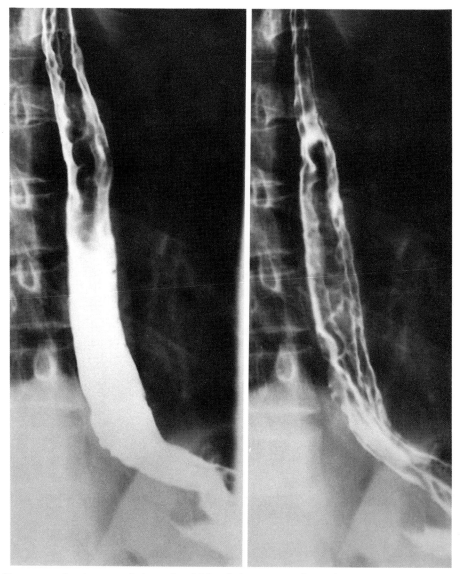

A. X-ray examination reveals irregular folds of the mucosa from the upper to middle esophagus. On a double contrast film a pearl-necklace sign is seen.

43

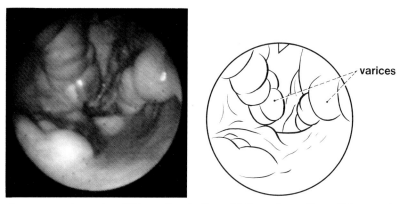

B. Esophagoscopy shows bead-like varices in the mid-thoracic portion of the esophagus.

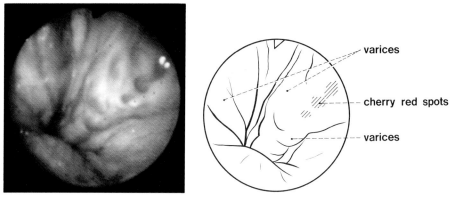

C. In the lower esophagus, dilatation of small vessels on the varices is observed (varices on varices).

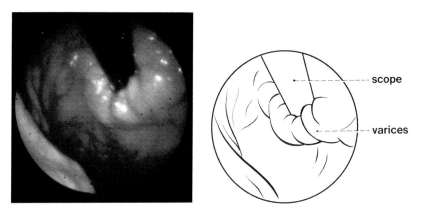

D. A retrograde view from the stomach showing the cardia with gastric varices around its orifice. No erosion is present in the esophagus or stomach.

Case 19   Achalasia

A 45-year-old female. *Chief complaint:* dysphagia for about ten years. When she is in good condition, she can eat solid foods without any difficulty but, in poor condition, even liquid foods pass poorly. Her symptoms do not significantly change. Laboratory data were normal.

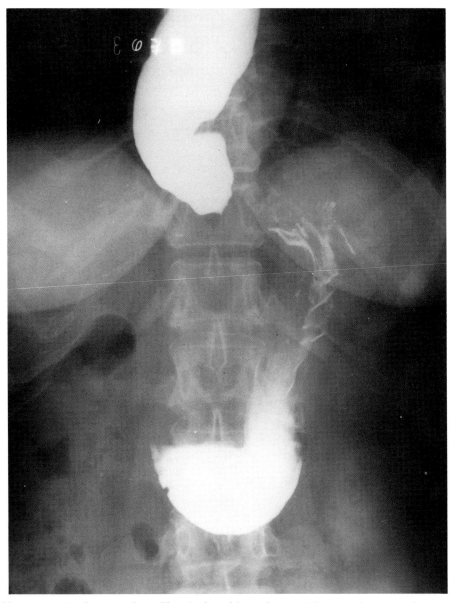

A. X-ray examination reveals a dilated, sigmoid esophagus with stenosis at the distal end of the esophagus. No gas is seen in the fornix of the stomach.

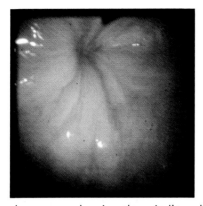
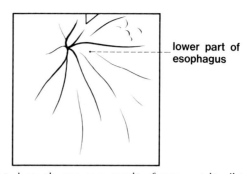

lower part of
esophagus

B. Esophagoscopy showing the winding, dilated esophagus as a result of spasm at its distal end. The mucosa appears normal (top).

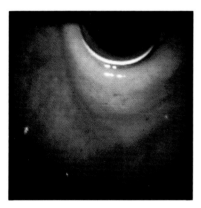
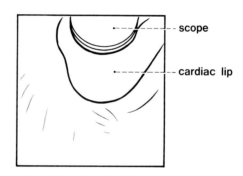

scope

cardiac lip

C. Endoscopic picture of the retrograde view from the stomach. The esophageal mucosa is seen, through the cardiac orifice, adjacent to the shaft of the scope. The gastric mucosa is also observed at the level of the abdominal esophagus and appears to roll up to the shaft of the scope.

Case 20   Reconstruction of the esophagus: stoma of an esophagojejunostomy

A 49-year-old female. *Chief complaint:* asymptomatic. One year earlier, a total gastrectomy was performed due to gastric cancer. Esophagojejunostomy (Roux-en-Y) was performed. She is asymptomatic at present. Laboratory data were normal.

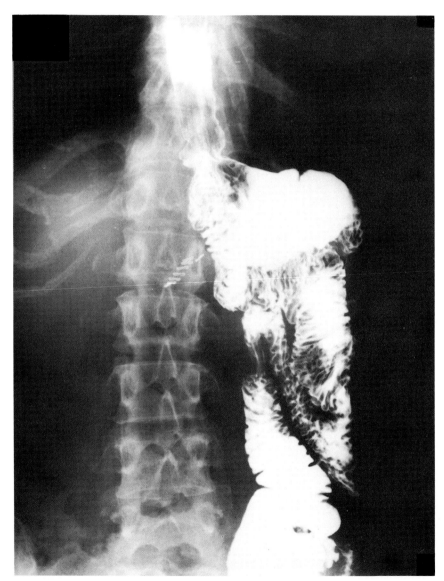

A. An X-ray of the esophagojejunostomy. The barium meal passes smoothly into the jejunum. No stenosis is seen.

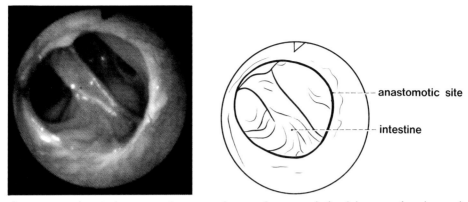

B. Esophagoscopy shows the stoma between the esophagus and the jejunum, the size and distensibility of which are apparently adequate. Post-operative esophagitis is not observed.

3

Endoscopy of the Stomach

TATSUZO KASUGAI, M.D.

Gastrofiberscopy (endoscopy of the stomach) is one of the most universal procedures among endoscopic examinations.

Indications and Contraindications

Endoscopy is indicated for patients suspected of having any kind of gastric disease such as acute and chronic gastritis, peptic ulcer, carcinoma, sarcoma, polyp, submucosal tumor, tuberculosis, syphilis, diverticulum, varices and others. Contraindications are described in Chaper 1.

Instruments

The forward-viewing and side-viewing fiberscopes are used for examination of the stomach (Figs. 3-1 to 3-3).

Taking color pictures or cine photography during the endoscopy is useful for interpretation of a lesion by other physicians, follow-up study, retrospective study and

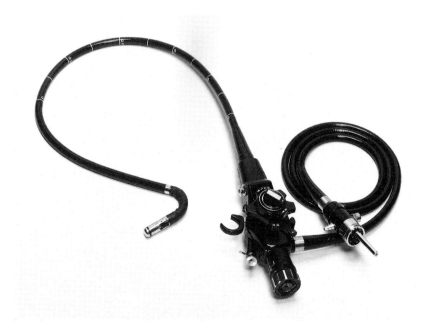

Fig. 3-1 Olympus gastrofiberscope GTF type B100 (side-viewing).

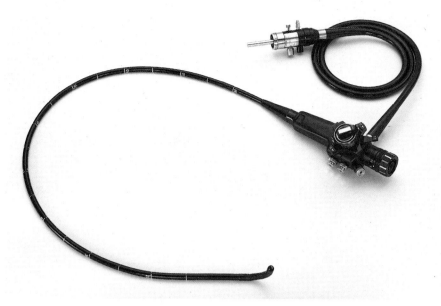

Fig. 3-2 Olympus panendoscope GIF type P3.

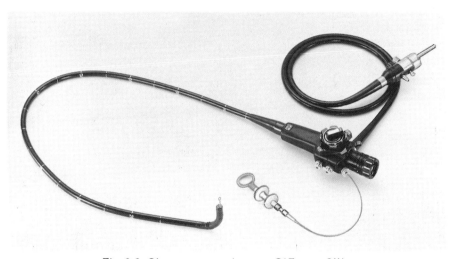

Fig. 3-3 Olympus panendoscope GIF type QW.

teaching. Color photographs are taken by a 35 m/m or 16 m/m special camera (sc-16-type 3) for a fiberscope attached to the eyepiece of the scope. The model GTF gastro-fiberscope has a tiny camera incorporated into the tip of the fiberscope with which very sharp color pictures are taken.

In the past different fiberscopes were used for photography, cytology and biopsy. However, newer models such as GTF type B100 satisfy multi-purposes, reducing discomfort and cost of examination for patients and saving time for physicians.

In cases in which malignancy.is suspected biopsy and brushing cytology under direct vision should be performed by such a gastrofiberscope as GTF type B100.

Technique

Gastrofiberscopy is performed with the patient in the left lateral decubitus position.

The tip of the scope is introduced beyond the root of the tongue through the naturally widely opened mouth to the pharynx where the tip is generally stopped with slight resistance. The tip of a side-viewing fiberscope is gently pushed in simultaneously with the patient's swallow and introduced into the esophagus. At this moment the tip of the scope should be inserted along the axis of the esophagus. If the tip is flexed downward, the left part of the wall of the pharynx might be injured.

The scope is passed through the gastric cardia with slight resistance about 40 to 45 cm from the incisors and enters the stomach at 45 to 50 cm.

A forward-viewing scope is introduced from the oral cavity into the esophagus under direct vision and passed through the esophagus and then forwarded into the stomach via the esophagogastric junction under vision.

The angulus, antrum, pylorus, lower, middle and upper body are observed and photographed by manipulation of the scope with the angle up and down, right and left. For observation of the cardia and fornix special maneuvers for U-turns and J-turns are used if necessary.

Observation of the entire lesion from a suitable distance and close-up observations are required to obtain details of a lesion.

Gastric Biopsy

Gastric biopsy is performed according to necessity.

The technique of gastric biopsy has advanced along with improvement of the scopes — both side-viewing and forward-viewing — and mucosal specimens can now be taken from anywhere within the stomach with the biopsy forceps without any blind area under direct vision.

Diagnostic accuracy by endoscopic biopsy was 98.5 percent in early gastric cancer and 93.1 percent in advanced gastric cancer in our department. The results of gastric biopsy under direct vision are shown in Table 3-1 and those of lavage cytology under direct vision in Table 3-2.

At present, by use of endoscopy it has become possible to detect any lesion of the stomach including even small lesions, 2 to 3 mm in diameter, and to obtain a histological diagnosis.

Biopsied specimens taken from a lesion suspected of being border-line or malignant endoscopically are evaluated according to histological grouping of biopsied materials from the stomach for diagnosis of gastric carcinoma (Table 3-3).

Table 3-1 Gastric biopsy in cancer of the stomach.
(Aichi Cancer Center Hospital, 1964 to 1974.)

	No. of patients	Positive	Accuracy (%)
Carcinoma	2,039	1,917	94.0
Early	336	331	98.5
Advanced	1,703	1,586	93.1
Sarcoma	21	10	47.6
Lymphoma	17	8	47.1
Leiomyosarcoma	3	1	33.3
Unclassified	1	1	100.0

Table 3-2 Results of gastric lavage cytology under direct vision †.

	No. of cases	+	±	—	Diagnostic accuracy (%)
Gastric cancer	512	494	7	11	96.0
Early Ca.	128	122	2	4	95.3
Advanced Ca.	384	372	5	7	96.9
Gastric sarcoma	10*	9*		1	90.0

*   Including 2 cases examined by imprint smear.
†   From Kasugai, T. and Kobayashi, S.: Evaluation of biopsy and cytology in the diagnosis of gastric cancer. Amer. J. Gastroenterol. 62: 199-203, 1974.

Table 3-3 Histological grouping of biopsied materials from the stomach for diagnosis of gastric carcinoma.

Group I.   Normal and benign lesion without atypia
Group II.   Benign lesion with slight atypia
Group III. Border-line lesion
Group IV. Lesion strongly suspected of carcinoma
Group V.   Carcinoma

Advanced Gastric Cancer

Advanced gastric cancers are classified into four types based on visual inspection of the mucosal surface of the lesion, according to Borrmann's classification (Fig. 3-4).

Early Gastric Cancer

Definition and classification of early carcinoma of the stomach have been agreed upon in Japan to facilitate discussions among radiologists, endoscopists, cytologists, surgeons, and pathologists who have been engaged in detection and study of gastric carcinoma. These definitions and classifications are widely adopted in Japan.

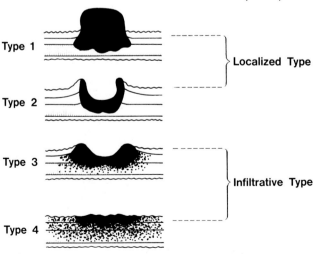

Fig. 3-4 Borrmann's classification of advanced gastric cancer. (From Japanese Research Society for Gastric Cancer: The general rules for the gastric cancer study in surgery and pathology. Jap. J. Surg. 11: 127-145, 1981.)

Definition of Early Carcinoma of the Stomach

At the annual meeting of the Japan Gastroenterological Endoscopy Society in 1962 and of the Japanese Research Society for Gastric Cancer in 1963, early gastric carcinoma was defined as carcinoma of the stomach in which carcinomatous invasion was limited to the mucosa and submucosa.

Macroscopic Classification of Early Gastric Carcinoma

Borrmann's classification of gastric carcinoma which is most widely used is based mainly on the difference in the form of submucosal invasion. Therefore, it is not applicable to the classification of early carcinoma whose invasion is limited to the mucosa and submucosa. To cope with this problem, a macroscopic classification for early carcinoma, shown in Figure 3-5, was proposed in 1962 by the Japan Gastroenterological Endoscopy Society. The classification has been widely adopted and has contributed greatly to the recent progress in the diagnosis of early carcinoma of the stomach.

Type I (Protruded Type)

    Protrusion into the gastric lumen is eminent.

Type II (Superficial Type)

    Unevenness of the surface is inconspicuous. This is further divided into three subtypes, i.e.

    Type IIa (Elevated Type)

        The surface is slightly elevated.

    Type IIb (Flat Type)

        Almost no recognizable elevation or depression from the surrounding mucosa.

    Type IIc (Depressed Type)

        The surface is slightly depressed.

Type III (Excavated Type)

    An excavation in the gastric wall is prominent.

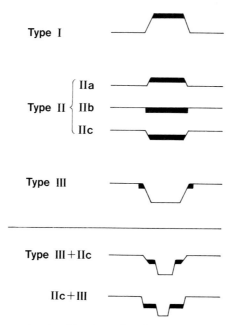

Fig. 3-5 Macroscopic classification of early gastric carcinoma proposed by the Japan Gastroenterological Endoscopy Society (1962).

In applying this classification, the histogenesis of carcinomas should not be considered. The difference between type IIc and type III is that the depression of the latter is limited beyond the submucosa.

When a lesion consists of diverse morphological patterns, two or more types are described in combination, e.g. type III+IIc or IIc+III. The first Roman numeral indicates the predominant pattern.

Prognosis of Early Gastric Cancer

Early gastric cancers have a much better prognosis than advanced ones. Honda reported a 10-year survival rate of 80.2 percent in 1,780 cases of early gastric cancer collected from major centers in Japan. We have a 5-year survival rate of 94.3 percent and a 10-year survival rate of 85.5 percent in early gastric cancer as shown in Table 3-4.

Table 3-4 Survival rate of gastric cancer after surgery. (Aichi Cancer Center Hospital, 1964 to 1976.)

		5 years %	10 years %
Early Ca.	419	94.3 (98.6)	85.5 (94.3)
Advanced Ca.	940	52.1 (53.4)	40.9 (46.3)
Total	1,359	65.1 (67.2)	54.7 (61.0)

(   ): Non-cancer death cases were excluded.

Elevated Lesion in the Stomach

Elevated lesions in the stomach are usually classified into four types: flat, sessile, semipedunculated and pedunculated, according to Yamada's classification as shown in Figure 3-6.

Complications and Precautions of Gastrofiberscopy

Gastrofiberscopy is, in general, a safe procedure, but there are some possible hazards.

Use of anticholinergic agents may aggravate glaucoma and hyperprostatism.

Problems from medication may occur after patients have left the hospital. Patients should not drive within several hours after the examination when a sedative has been given, because the effects of various sedatives are usually prolonged.

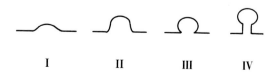

I   II   III   IV

Fig. 3-6 Macroscopic classification of elevated lesions of the stomach (Yamada's classification). (From Yamada, T. and Fukutomi, H.: Elevated lesion of the stomach. I to Cho (Stomach & Intestine) 1: 145-150, 1966.)

Perforation may occur in the pharynx and cervical esophagus and cardia where the fiberscope is usually passed blindly, especially in cases in which these sites are distorted or diseased.

Imprudent force is usually responsible for perforation.

Although surgical advice should always be sought immediately in cases with a suspicion of perforation, many cases can be treated conservatively with a regimen consisting of drainage, intravenous feeding and antibiotics.

The tip of a flexible endoscope can actually impact in a hiatus hernia or the distal esophagus during the U-turn method (retroversion maneuver). Blind and forceful withdrawal should not be attempted if impaction is suspected. Disimpaction is best achieved by advancing the instrument.

Gastrofiberscopy like other instrumental procedures sometimes induces cardiac dysrhythmias. Cardiographic monitoring is advisable when endoscopy is performed in patients with serious cardiac disability. Full resuscitation equipment must always be available.

Transmission of infection is rarely documented. Bacterial contamination will not occur if endoscopes are properly cleaned and disinfected at the time of each procedure, but they cannot be previously sterilized. Viral transmission is very difficult to document and to prevent. The endoscopic procedure and precautions in patients with a positive hepatitis associated antigen are described in the indications and contraindications of Chapter 1.

In general, the most effective way to avoid complications in endoscopy is a carefully performed procedure.

Acute Upper Gastrointestinal Hemorrhage

In cases with acute upper gastrointestinal hemorrhage, endoscopy should be performed by a skilled endoscopist within a few hours of admission, using a forward-viewing fiberscope that permits visualization of the esophagus, stomach and duodenum (panendoscope, e.g. GIF type P3 shown in Fig. 3-2 or GIF type QW shown in Fig. 3-3).

Dye Scattering Method

A dye scattering method can be carried out by the gastroscope to delineate the extent of a lesion and to help differentiate between malignant and benign lesions.

Endoscopic Surgery

Endoscopic surgery such as polypectomy, using a snare cautery wire (Fig. 3-7) introduced through a biopsy channel of a gastrofiberscope, and special coagulation device to prevent bleeding, is now an established procedure.

Laser Endoscopy

Endoscopic Nd:YAG laser irradiation for control of acute gastrointestinal bleeding has been performed, and also endoscopic YAG laser treatment has been successfully attempted in patients with types IIa and IIc early gastric cancer and the protruded type of border-line lesion of the stomach (Fig. 3-8).

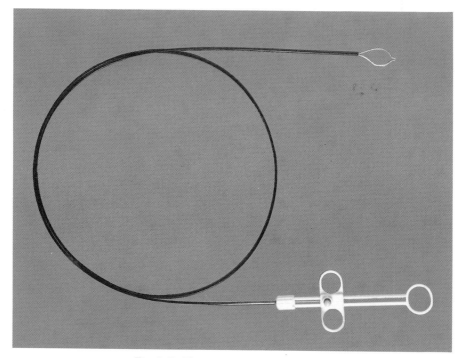

Fig. 3-7 Olympus snare cautery wire.

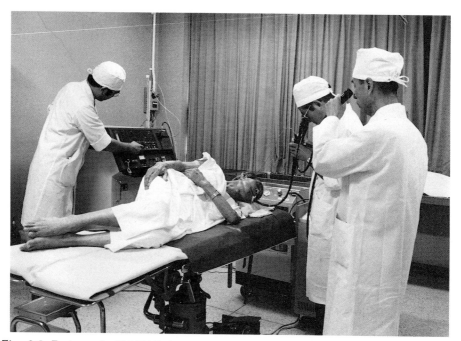

Fig. 3-8 Endoscopic Nd:YAG laser treatment in a patient with early gastric cancer is performed.

REFERENCES

1) Borrmann, R.: Geschwülste des Magens und Duodenums. In: Henke, F. and Lubarsch, O. (eds.) Handbuch der Speziellen Pathologischen Anatomie und Histologie, Vol. 4, Part 1, pp. 812-1054, J. Springer, Berlin, 1926.

2) Cotton, P.B.: Complications and precautions. In: Cotton, P.B., and Williams, C.B. (eds.) Practical Gastrointestinal Endoscopy, pp. 42-44, Blackwell, Oxford, 1980.

3) Frühmorgen, P., Bodem, F., Reidenback, H.D., Kaduk, B., and Demling, L.: Endoscopic laser coagulation of bleeding gastrointestinal lesions with report of the first therapeutic application in man. Gastrointest. Endosc. 23: 73-75, 1976.

4) Honda, T.: A ten year-long term results of early gastric cancer. Gastroenterol. Endosc. 19: 613-629, 1977. (in Japanese)

5) Ito, Y., Sugiura, H., Tanehiro, K., Kasugai, T., and Hanawa, K.: Endoscopic applications of the Nd: YAG laser. J. Jap. Soc. Laser Med. 1: 393-399, 1980. (in Japanese)

6) Japanese Research Society for Gastric Cancer: The general rules for the gastric cancer study in surgery and pathology. Jap. J. Surg. 11: 127-145, 1981.

7) Kasugai, T.: Gastric biopsy under direct vision by the fibergastroscope. Gastrointest. Endosc. 15: 33-39, 1968.

8) Kasugai, T. and Kobayashi, S.: Evaluation of biopsy and cytology in the diagnosis of gastric cancer. Amer. J. Gastroenterol. 62: 199-203, 1974.

9) Kasugai, T.: The role of endoscopy in the diagnosis of gastrointestinal disease. In: Powell, L.W. and Piper, D.W. (eds.) Fundamentals of Gastroenterology, 3rd ed., pp. 148-154, ADIS Press, Sydney, 1980.

10) Nagayo, T., Mochizuki, T., Sano, R., and Sugano, H.: A draft for histological grouping of biopsied materials of the stomach for diagnosis of gastric carcinoma. Gan no Rinsho (Jap. J. Cancer Clinics) 15: 937-952, 1969. (in Japanese)

11) Yamada, T. and Fukutomi, H.: Elevated lesion of the stomach. I to Cho (Stomach & Intestine) 1: 145-150, 1966. (in Japanese)

Case 1   Normal gastric mucosa

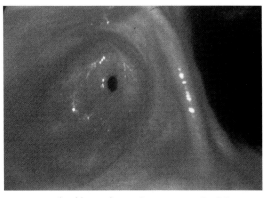
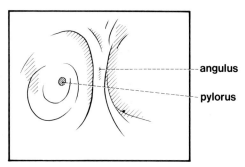

A. Normal gastric antrum of a 35-year-old male complaining of epigastric pain.

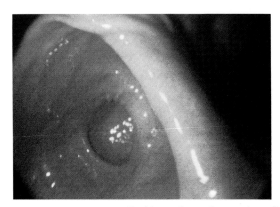
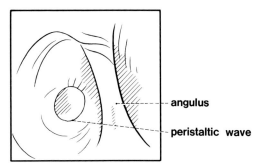

B. Normal gastric angulus of the same patient as Figure A.

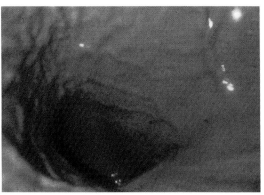
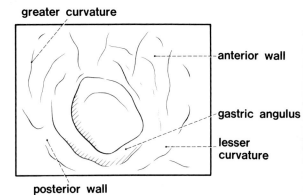

C. Normal gastric body of a 26-year-old female complaining of epigastric pain.

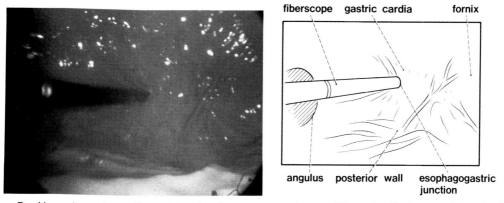

D. Normal gastric cardia and fornix of the same patient as Figure C. Endoscopy taken by U-turn method.

Case 2   Chronic superficial gastritis

A 51-year-old male. *Chief complaint:* epigastric pain.

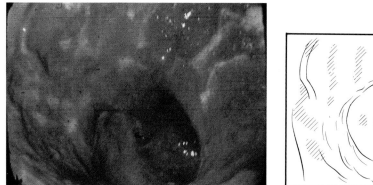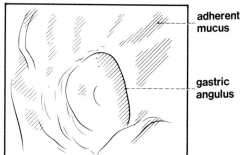

Endoscopy showing the gastric mucosa of the lower body with adherent mucus.

Case 3   Chronic superficial gastritis

A 20-year-old female. *Chief complaints:* nausea and belching in the fasting period.

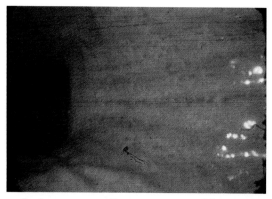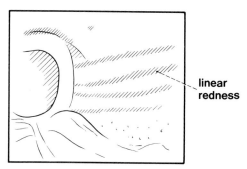

Endoscopy revealing many areas of linear redness called "Kammrötung" in the gastric body especially on the lesser curvature.

Case 4 Chronic atrophic gastritis

A 61-year-old male. *Chief complaint:* epigastric fullness.

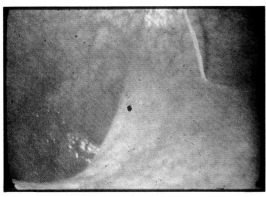 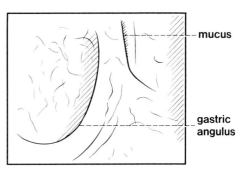

Endoscopy revealing transparent blood vessels in the submucosal layer of the gastric body and antrum.

Case 5 Chronic atrophic hyperplastic gastritis

A 60-year-old female. *Chief complaint:* anorexia.

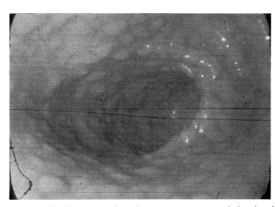 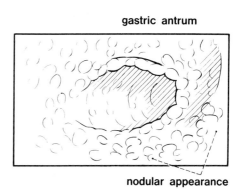

Endoscopy showing numerous nodules in the antrum and lower body of the stomach.

Case 6   Chronic hypertrophic gastritis

A 40-year-old male. *Chief complaint:* epigastric pain in the fasting period and at night.

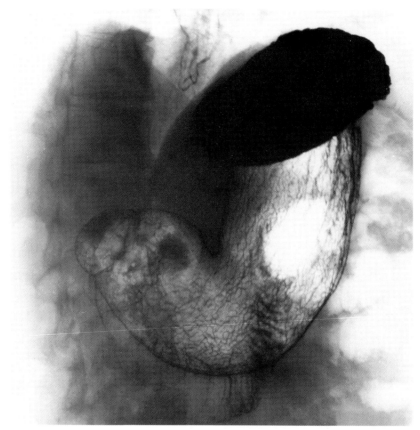

A. Barium meal examination (double contrast method) showing a cobblestone appearance of the gastric mucosa.

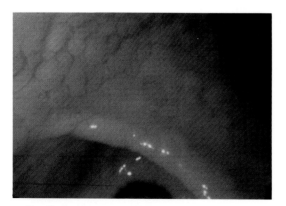
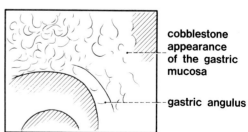

cobblestone
appearance
of the gastric
mucosa

gastric angulus

B. Endoscopy revealing a cobblestone appearance of the mucosa of the lower gastric body, especially on the anterior wall.

63

Case 7 Erosive gastritis

A 30-year-old male. *Chief complaint:* epigastric pain.

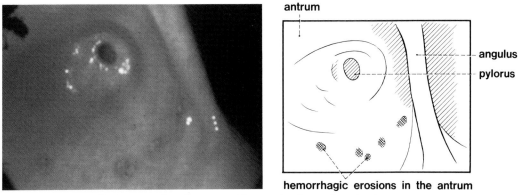

Endoscopy showing several hemorrhagic erosions in the antrum.

Case 8 Acute gastritis

A 42-year-old male. *Chief complaints:* epigastric pain and nausea.

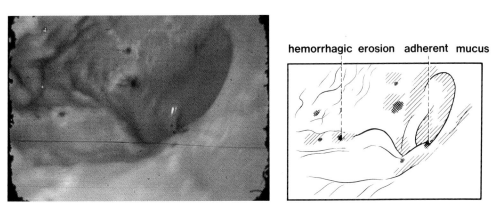

Endoscopy revealing many hemorrhagic erosions in the gastric mucosa covered with adherent mucus of the antrum and lower body.

Case 9　Verrucous erosive gastritis

A 46-year-old male. *Chief complaint:* epigastric pain.

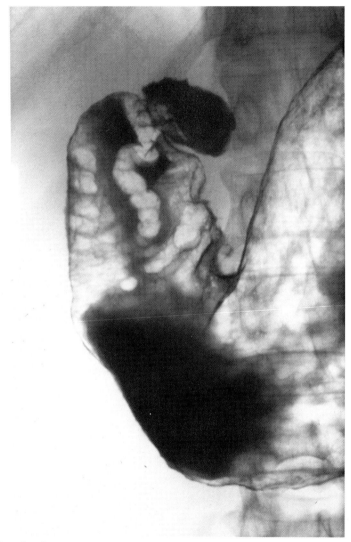

A. Upper GI series shows green caterpillar-like elevations and nodular elevations in the antrum.

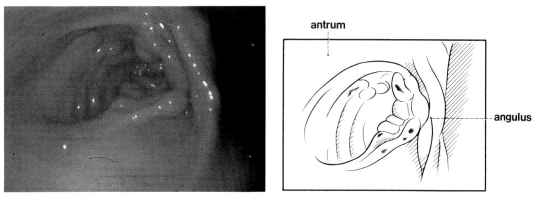

B. There are many, small, flat elevations with a central erosion in the antrum.

Case 10   Open gastric ulcer

A 44-year-old male. *Chief complaint:* epigastric pain.

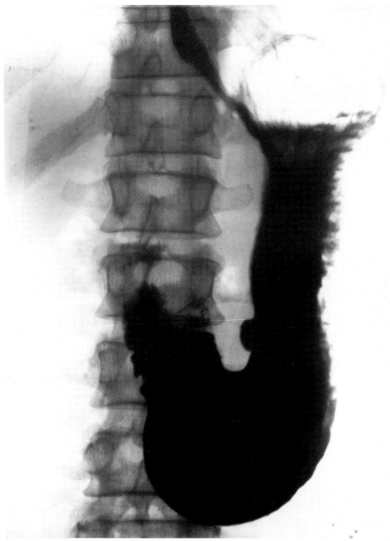

A. Barium meal examination revealing a huge niche on the lesser curvature of the lower body of the stomach.

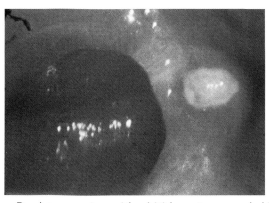 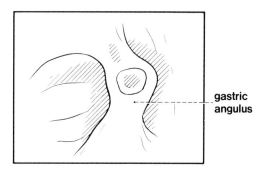

B. An open ulcer with whitish coat surrounded by edematous ulcer margins is visualized on the lesser curvature of the lower body of the stomach.

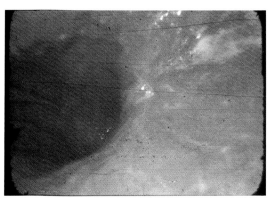 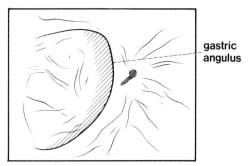

C. Healing stage, examined one month after the first examination. An irregularly shaped healing ulcer with converging folds is visualized on the lesser curvature of the lower body of the stomach.

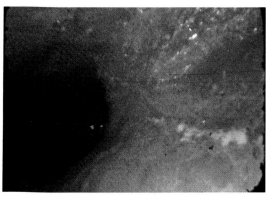 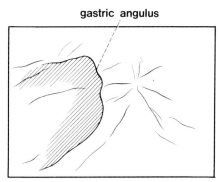

D. Healed stage, ulcer scar, examined two months after the first endoscopy. A gastric ulcer scar with converging folds is seen on the lesser curvature of the lower body of the stomach.

Case 11   Active gastric ulcer

A 46-year-old male. *Chief complaints:* fasting epigastric pain and vomiting. *Treatment:* partial gastrectomy.

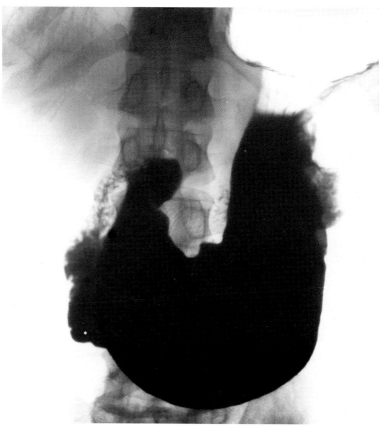

A. Barium meal examination revealing a huge niche at the angulus and in the deformed duodenal bulb.

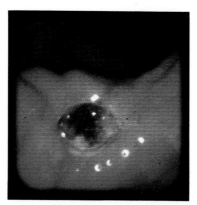 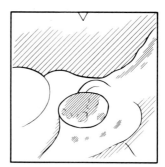

B. Endoscopy performed with a gastrointestinal fiberscope GIF type Q reveals a huge, deep ulcer, the floor of which is covered with a yellowish black coat at the angulus.

Case 12 Active gastric ulcer

A 27-year-old male. *Chief complaint:* epigastric pain. *Treatment:* medical treatment.

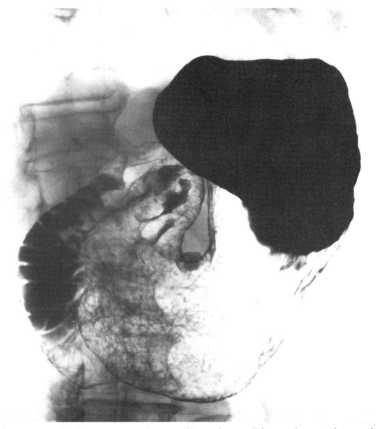

A. Double contrast barium meal study revealing a huge niche at the gastric angulus.

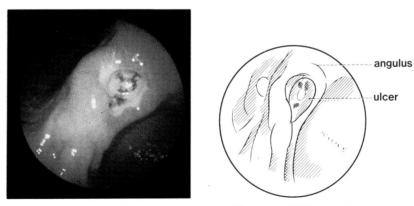

B. Endoscopy performed with a gastrointestinal fiberscope GIF type Q reveals a hugé, deep ulcer, the floor of which is covered with a yellowish white coat with some bloody spots, surrounded by edematous, thick ulcer margins at the gastric angulus.

Case 13   Gastric ulcer scar

A 43-year-old female. *Chief complaint:* asymptomatic.

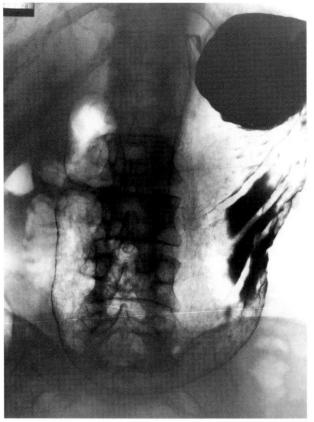

A. Barium meal examination (double contrast method) shows an ulcer scar with converging folds on the posterior wall of the lower body of the stomach.

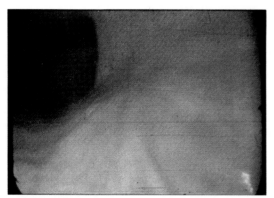 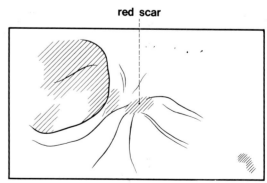

B. A red scar with converging folds is visualized on the lesser curvature aspect of the posterior wall of the lower body of the stomach.

Case 14 **Kissing ulcer**

A 43-year-old male. *Chief complaints:* tarry stool and epigastric pain.

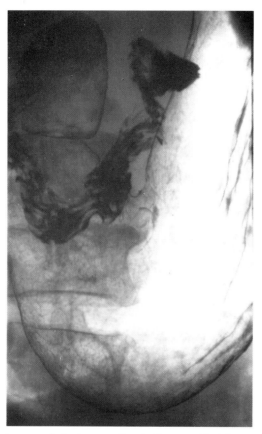

A. Double contrast barium meal study revealing both a small niche on the anterior aspect of the angulus and a niche of medium size with several converging folds on the posterior wall of the lower body of the stomach.

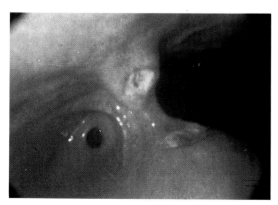 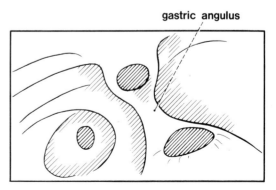

B. Two open ulcers with edematous walls are respectively visualized on the anterior and posterior aspects of the gastric angulus.

Case 15   Multiple ulcer

A 62-year-old male. *Chief complaint:* epigastric discomfort in the fasting period.

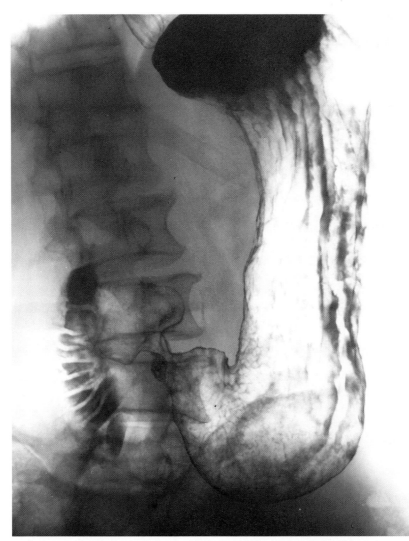

A. Barium meal examination showing multiple tiny niches on the lesser curvature of the lower body and deformed antrum with shortening of the lesser curvature, and the deformed duodenal bulb.

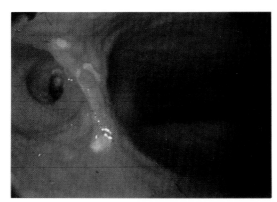 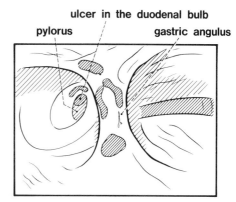

pylorus   ulcer in the duodenal bulb   gastric angulus

B. Many irregularly shaped ulcers are visualized on the angulus area and the prepyloric area. A duodenal ulcer is also seen through the pylorus.

Case 16   Penetrating ulcer

A 56-year-old male. *Chief complaints:* tarry stool and epigastric pain.

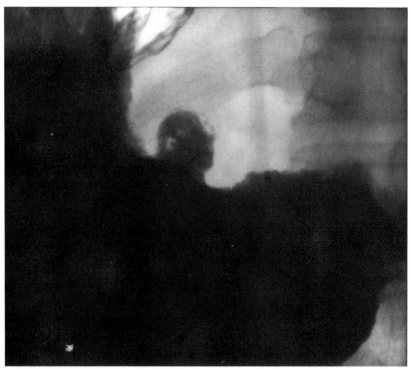

A. Barium meal study with patient in the prone position showing a huge niche with air bubbles at the gastric angulus.

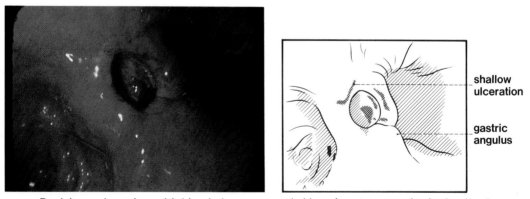

B. A huge, deep ulcer with bloody base surrounded by edematous margins is visualized.

Case 17   **Linear ulcer**

A 47-year-old male. *Chief complaint:* epigastric pain.

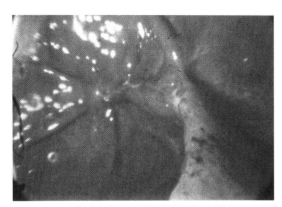 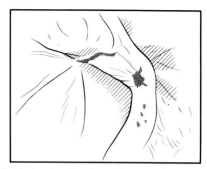

An irregularly shaped linear ulcer with converging folds is visualized on the anterior aspect of the gastric angulus.

Case 18   Advanced gastric cancer : Borrmann's type 1

A 70-year-old female. *Chief complaint:* epigastric pain.

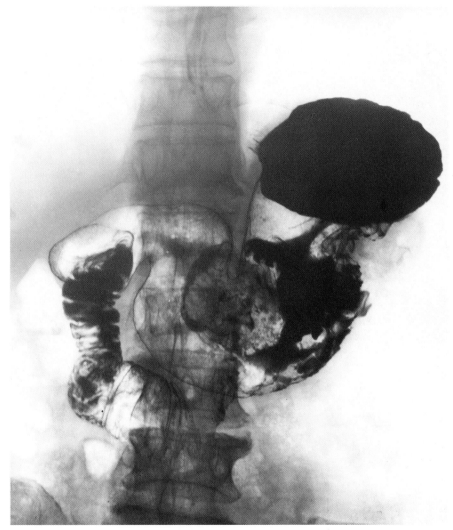

A. Barium meal examination revealing a huge tumor in the lower body and proximal antrum of the stomach.

77

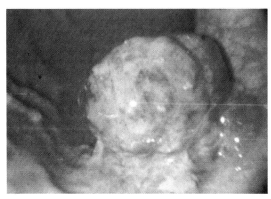
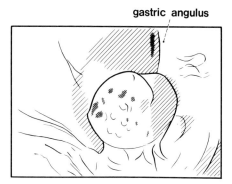

gastric angulus

B. Endoscopy showing a huge tumor with a nodular surface on the posterior aspect of the lower body of the stomach.

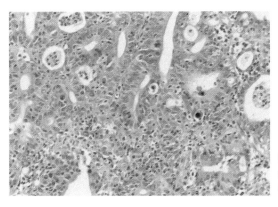

C. Histology of a biopsy specimen demonstrating a well-differentiated tubular adenocarcinoma. H.E., x 200

Case 19 Advanced gastric cancer : Borrmann's type 2

A 49-year-old male. *Chief complaint:* epigastric pain in the fasting period. *Treatment:* surgery was not done due to distant metastasis.

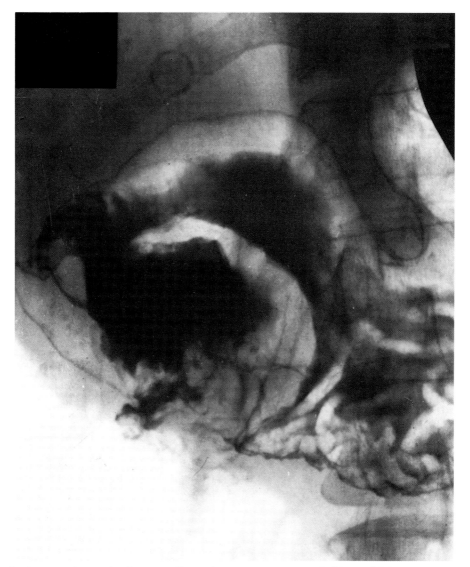

A. Barium meal examination revealing a huge crater surrounded by a thick embankment in the antrum.

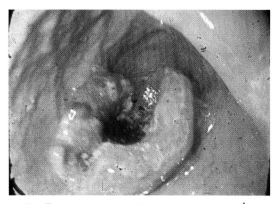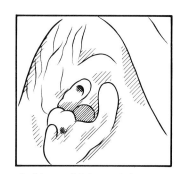

B. Endoscopy revealing a huge, deep crater surrounded by a thick, nodular crater wall on the posterior wall of the antrum.

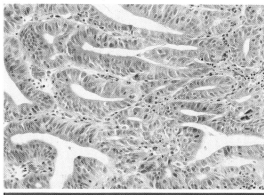

C. Biopsy demonstrates a moderately differentiated (papillo-) tubular adenocarcinoma. H.E., x 200

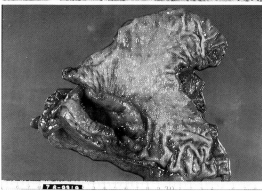

D. A huge crater surrounded by a crater wall is seen in a surgically resected specimen.

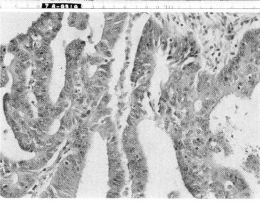

E. Histology of the surgically resected specimen demonstrating a well-differentiated tubular adenocarcinoma. H.E., x 200

Case 20   Advanced gastric cancer : Borrmann's type 3

A 78-year-old female. *Chief complaint:* epigastric pain. *Treatment:* gastrectomy was not performed because of distant metastasis and gastrojejunostomy was performed for pyloric stenosis.

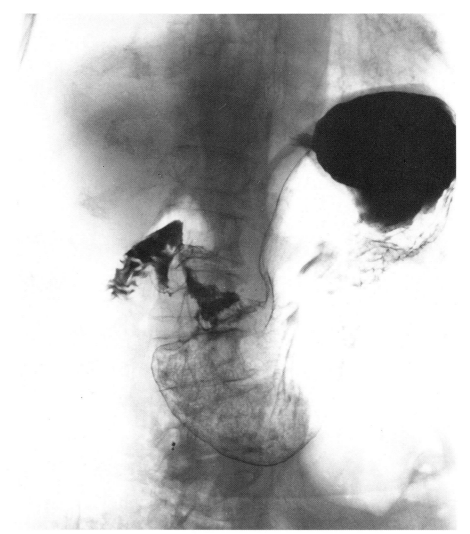

A. Barium meal study revealing a filling defect with an irregularly shaped ulcer crater in the gastric antrum, and findings of pyloric stenosis.

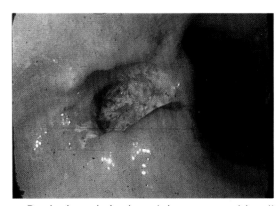 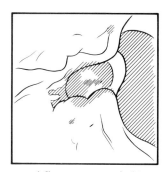

B. An irregularly shaped, huge crater with a dirty, rugged floor, surrounded by a thick nodular wall and tumor is visualized in the antrum.

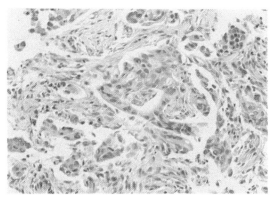

C. Biopsy shows a moderately differentiated tubular adenocarcinoma. H.E., x 200

Case 21   Advanced gastric cancer : Borrmann's type 3

A 48-year-old male.   *Chief complaint:* full sensation in the epigastrium.   *Treatment:* partial gastric resection.

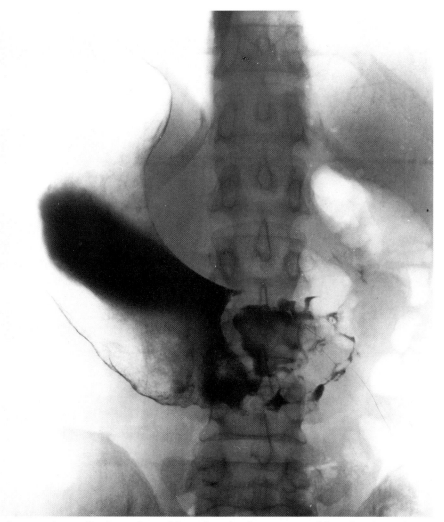

A. Barium meal examination taken with patient in the prone position showing a huge crater with embankment in the antrum.

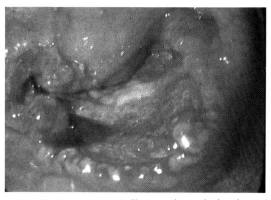 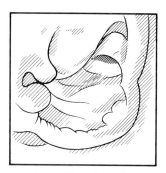

B. Endoscopy revealing an irregularly shaped huge crater with a bloody, uneven floor, surrounded by a thick nodular embankment and tumor in the antrum.

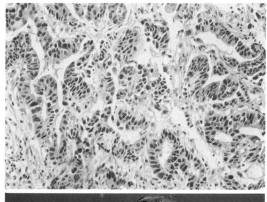

C. Biopsy demonstrates a moderately differentiated tubular adenocarcinoma. H.E., x200

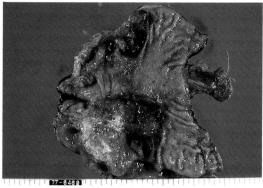

D. A huge crater is visualized in the antrum of a surgically resected specimen.

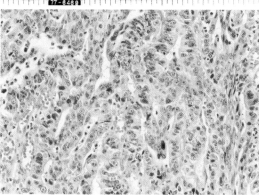

E. Histology of the surgically resected specimen demonstrates a moderately differentiated tubular adenocarcinoma. H.E., x 200

Case 22   Advanced gastric cancer : Borrmann's type 4

A 30-year-old male.   *Chief complaints:* fullness in the epigastrium and weight loss.
Treatment: total gastrectomy with splenectomy and esophagojejunostomy.

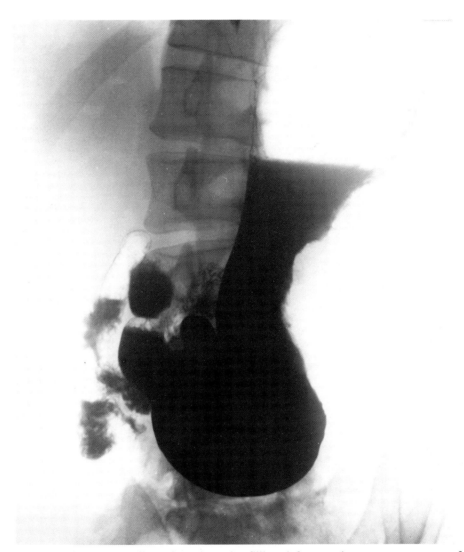

A. Barium meal study revealing a large irregular filling defect on the greater curvature of the
gastric body.

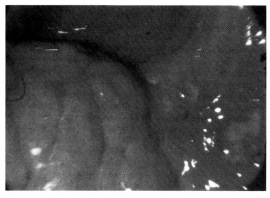

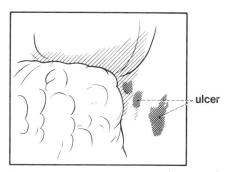

- ulcer

B. An aggregation of tumorous folds and irregularly shaped ulcers are seen on the posterior wall of the lower body of the stomach.

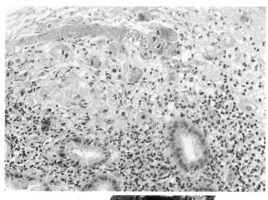

C. Biopsy demonstrates a signet ring cell (somewhat large in size) carcinoma. H.E. + Alcian-blue, x 200

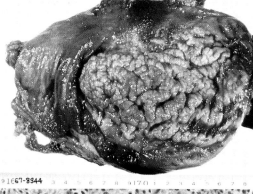

D. Surgically resected specimen shows numerous giant folds and irregularly shaped ulcers.

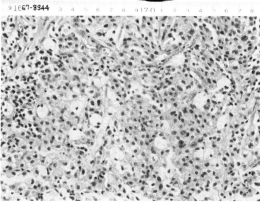

E. Histology of the surgically resected specimen demonstrating the signet ring cell carcinoma. H.E., x 200

Case 23   Advanced gastric cancer : Borrmann's type 4

A 57-year-old female. *Chief complaint:* poor appetite. *Treatment:* total gastrectomy with splenectomy and resection of the pancreatic tail.

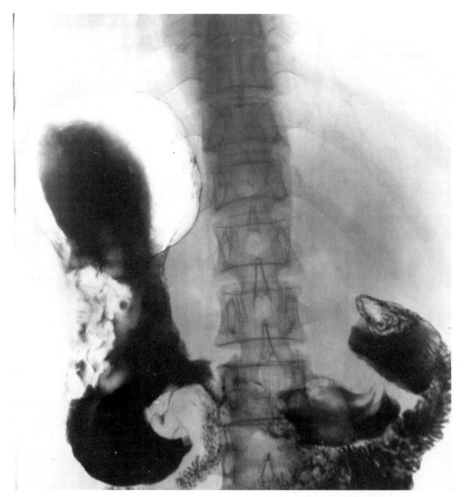

A. Barium meal study with patient in the prone position revealing irregular filling defects in the mid and lower body, and in the proximal antrum.

87

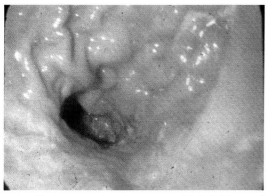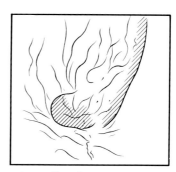

B. Endoscopy showing many thick folds on the anterior wall and greater curvature of the mid and lower body of the stomach and rigidity of the lesser curvature and posterior wall.

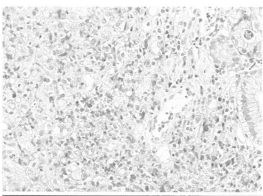

C. Biopsy specimen demonstrates a poorly differentiated adenocarcinoma. H.E., x 200

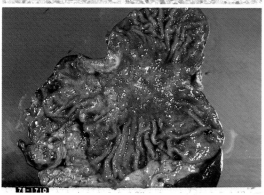

D. Surgically resected specimen shows many thick folds.

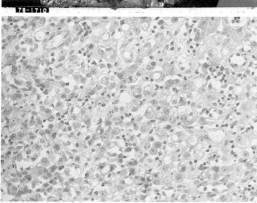

E. Histology demonstrates a poorly differentiated adenocarcinoma. H.E., x 200

Case 24   Early gastric cancer : type I

A 61-year-old male.   *Chief complaint:* upper abdominal pain.   *Treatment:* partial gastrectomy.

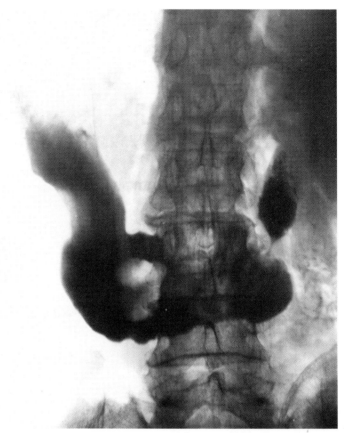

A. Barium meal study taken with patient in the prone position showing an oval filling defect on the anterior wall in the lower body of the stomach.

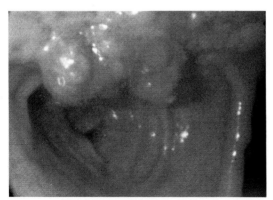
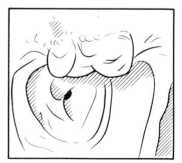

B. Endoscopy revealing an irregularly shaped tumor with a nodular surface on the anterior wall of the lower gastric body.
Gastric lavage cytology under direct vision by the fiberscope demonstrated cancer cells.

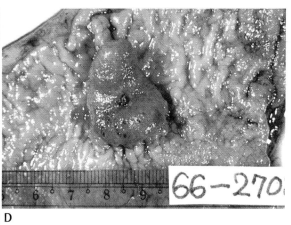

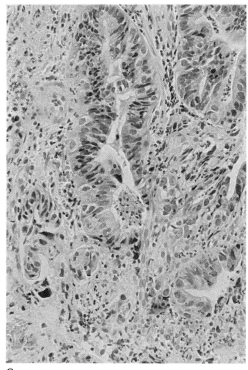

C. Histology of biopsy specimen demonstrates a tubular adenocarcinoma. H.E., x 200

D. Surgically resected specimen shows a polypoid tumor, 3.0 x 2.3 cm in diameter, on the anterior wall of the lower gastric body.

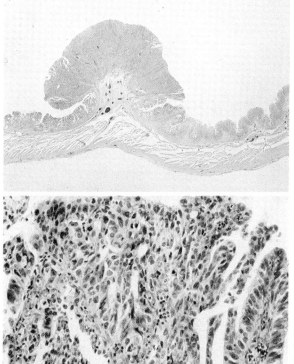

E. Low power histology of the surgically resected specimen shows a polypoid tumor.

F. Histology demonstrates a tubular adeno-carcinoma invading the mucosal and sub-mucosal layers. Lymph node metastases were found in one of 12 examined nodes. H.E., x 200

Case 25   Early gastric cancer : type I

A 64-year-old male.   *Chief complaint:* discomfort in the epigastrium.   *Treatment:* partial gastrectomy.

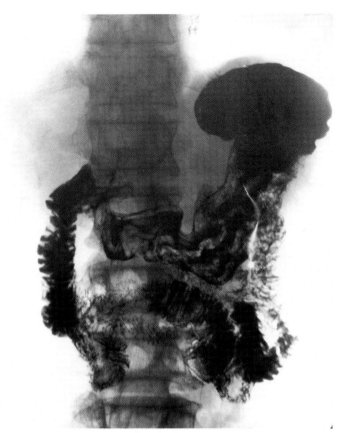

A. Barium meal study showing an oval filling defect on the posterior wall in the antrum.

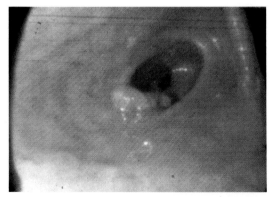 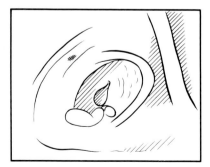

B. Endoscopy revealing a flat, green caterpillar-like elevation on the posterior wall in the distal antrum.
Gastric lavage cytology under direct vision by the fiberscope demonstrated cancer cells.

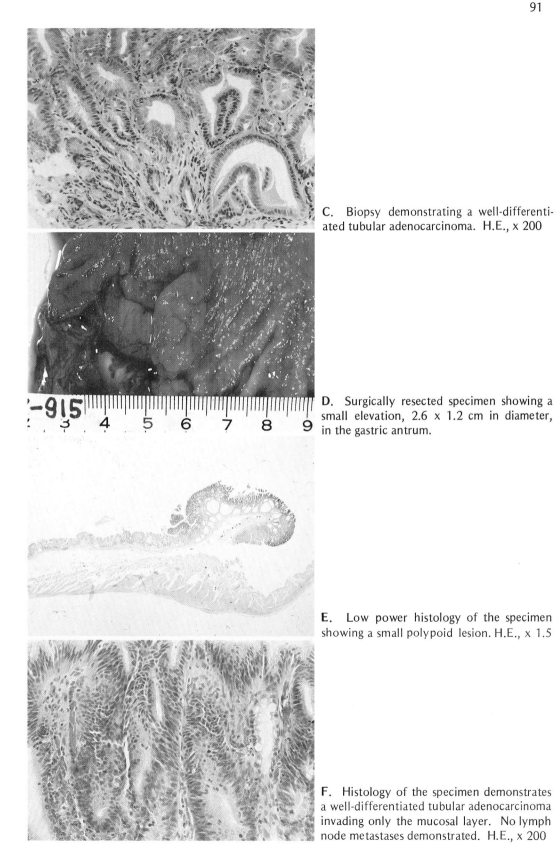

C. Biopsy demonstrating a well-differenti-ated tubular adenocarcinoma. H.E., x 200

D. Surgically resected specimen showing a small elevation, 2.6 x 1.2 cm in diameter, in the gastric antrum.

E. Low power histology of the specimen showing a small polypoid lesion. H.E., x 1.5

F. Histology of the specimen demonstrates a well-differentiated tubular adenocarcinoma invading only the mucosal layer. No lymph node metastases demonstrated. H.E., x 200

Case 26   Early gastric cancer : type IIa

A 54-year-old male. *Chief complaint:* epigastric pain. *Treatment:* partial gastrectomy.

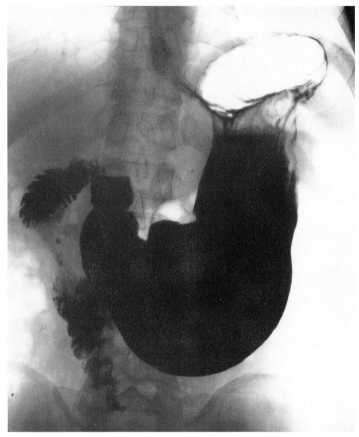

A. Barium meal examination showing a small filling defect on the lesser curvature of the lower gastric body close to the gastric angulus.

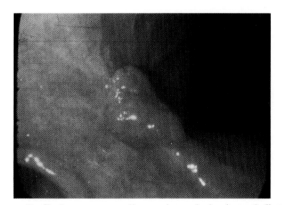
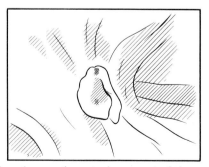

B. Endoscopy revealing an irregularly shaped, flat elevation on the anterior aspect of the gastric angulus.

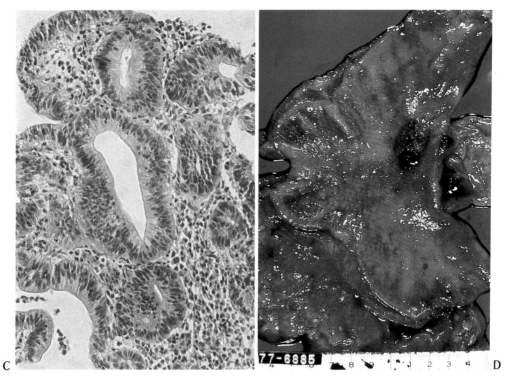

C. Biopsy demonstrating atypical cells, group IV – probably cancer cells. H.E., x 200

D. Surgically resected specimen shows a small polypoid tumor, 2.5 x 1.8 x 1.5 cm in size, on the anterior aspect of the lesser curvature of the lower gastric body.

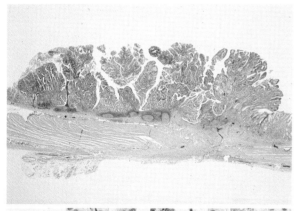

E. Low power histology of the specimen showing a polypoid lesion. H.E, x 1.5

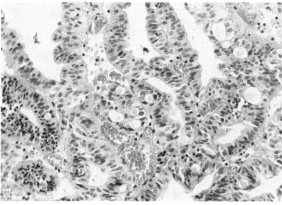

F. Histology of the specimen demonstrates a well-differentiated tubular adenocarcinoma invading the mucosal and submucosal layers. No lymph node metastases demonstrated. H.E., x 200

Case 27   **Early gastric cancer : type IIc**

A 49-year-old male. *Chief complaint:* asymptomatic. Screened on a gastric mass survey as probably having a lesion in the stomach. *Treatment:* partial gastrectomy.

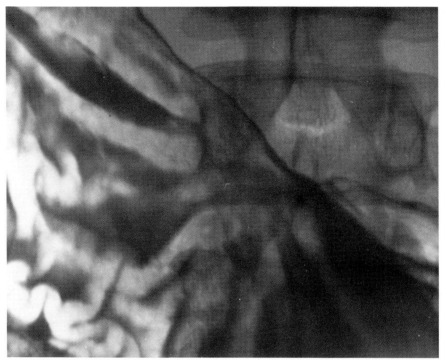

A. A barium meal examination taken with patient in the prone position revealing an irregularly shaped shallow ulceration with converging folds, tips of which show clubbing or thinning, on the anterior aspect of the lower gastric body.

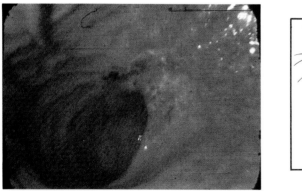 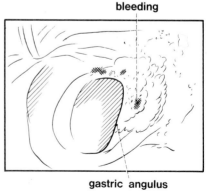

B. Endoscopy revealing an irregularly shaped shallow depression, in which there are many bleeding spots, with some converging folds on the anterior aspect of the lower gastric body.

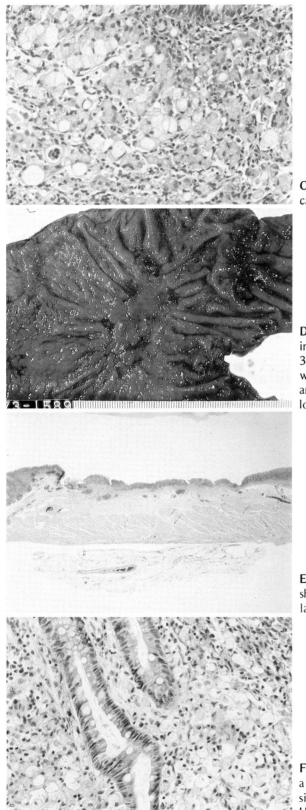

C. Biopsy demonstrating a signet ring cell carcinoma. H.E., x 200

D. Surgically resected specimen shows an irregularly shaped shallow ulceration, 5.5 x 3.0 cm in size, with converging folds, tips of which show clubbing or thinning, on the anterior aspect of the lesser curvature of the lower body of the stomach.

E. Low power histology of the specimen showing a shallow depression in the mucosal layer. H.E., x 1.5

F. Histology of the specimen demonstrating a signet ring cell carcinoma, in which invasion is limited only within the mucosal layer. H.E., x 200

Case 28   **Early gastric cancer : type IIc**

A 40-year-old female. *Chief complaint:* epigastric pain. *Treatment:* partial gastrectomy.

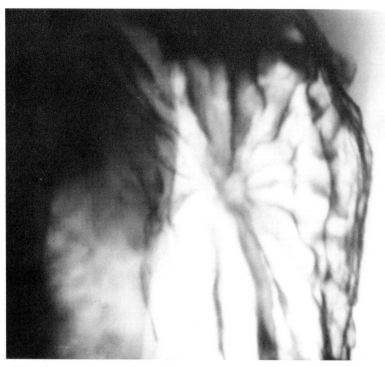

A. Upper GI series revealing an irregularly shaped ulceration with converging folds, tips of which show clubbing or thinning, on the anterior aspect of the greater curvature of the mid-body of the stomach.

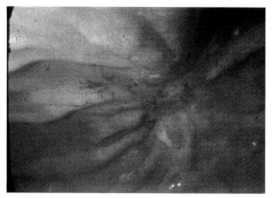 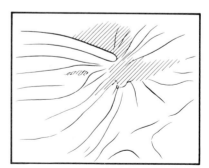

B. Endoscopy revealing an irregularly shaped shallow depression with converging folds, tips of which show thinning or clubbing, on the anterior aspect of the greater curvature of the mid gastric body.

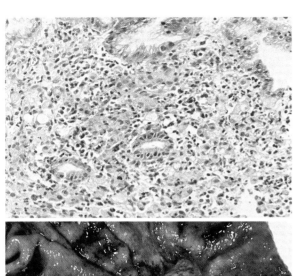

C. Biopsy demonstrating a tubular adeno-carcinoma. H.E., x 200

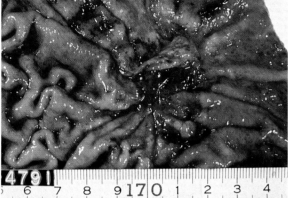

D. Surgically resected specimen shows an irregularly shaped shallow depression, 14.5 x 4 cm in diameter, with converging folds, tips of which show thinning or clubbing, on the anterior aspect of the greater curvature of the mid-body of the stomach.

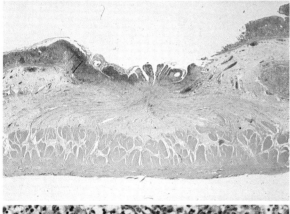

E. Low power histology shows a shallow ul-ceration in the mucosa. H.E., x 1.5

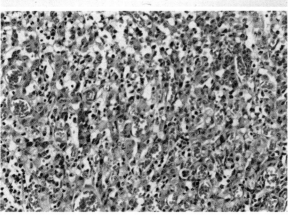

F. Histology of the specimen demonstrates a tubular adenocarcinoma invading only the mucosal layer. H.E., x 200

Case 29   Early gastric cancer : type IIc + III

A 63-year-old male. *Chief complaint:* dull pain in the epigastrium. *Treatment:* partial gastrectomy.

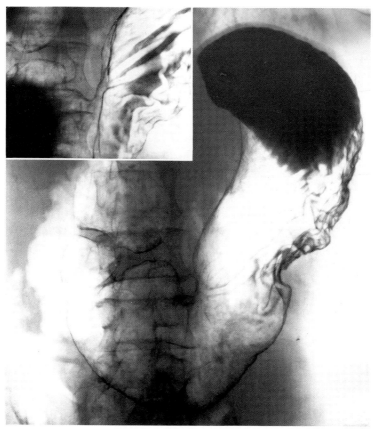

A. Barium meal examination showing an irregularly shaped, shallow ulceration with converging folds, tips of which show thinning at the angulus.

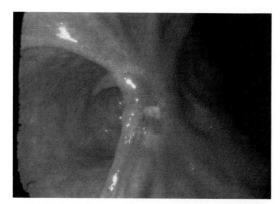 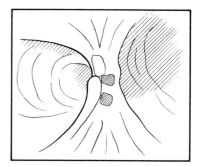

B. Endoscopy revealing a shallow depression with an irregularly shaped central ulceration and with converging folds, tips of which show thinning or clubbing on the gastric angulus.

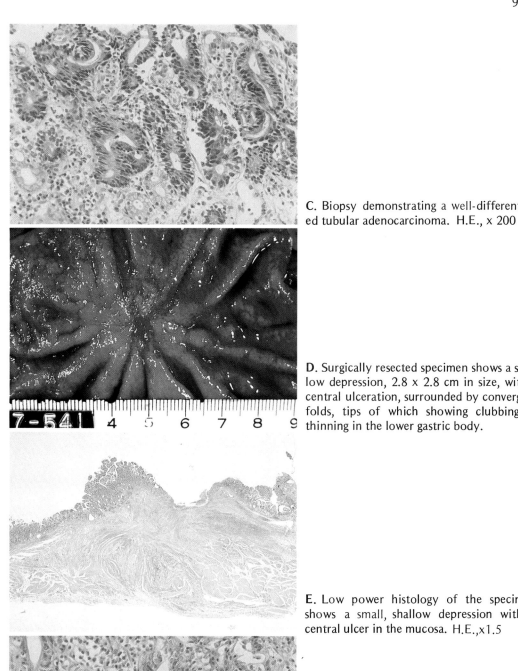

C. Biopsy demonstrating a well-differentiated tubular adenocarcinoma. H.E., x 200

D. Surgically resected specimen shows a shallow depression, 2.8 x 2.8 cm in size, with a central ulceration, surrounded by converging folds, tips of which showing clubbing or thinning in the lower gastric body.

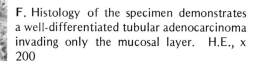

E. Low power histology of the specimen shows a small, shallow depression with a central ulcer in the mucosa. H.E.,x1.5

F. Histology of the specimen demonstrates a well-differentiated tubular adenocarcinoma invading only the mucosal layer. H.E., x 200

Case 30   Early gastric cancer : type IIc + III

A 51-year-old male. *Chief complaint:* epigastric pain. *Treatment:* partial gastrectomy.

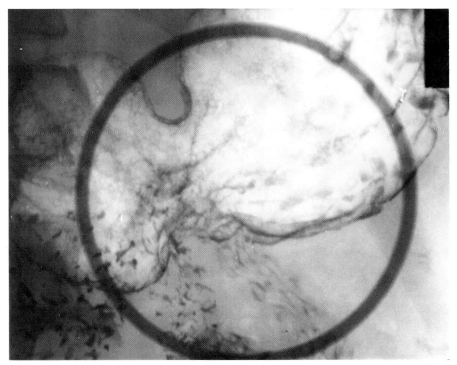

A. A barium meal study revealing an irregularly shaped depression with converging folds, tips of which show clubbing or thinning, on the greater curvature of the lower gastric body.

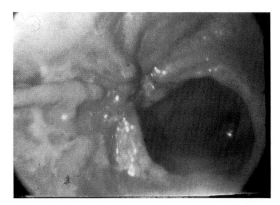
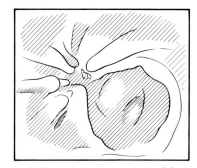

B. Endoscopic picture representing an irregularly shaped, shallow depression with converging folds which are clubbed and thinned at their tips on the anterior aspect of the greater curvature of the lower body.

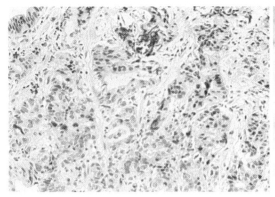

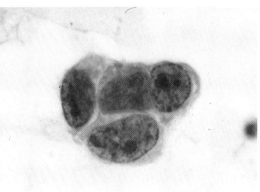

C. Biopsy demonstrates a moderately differentiated tubular adenocarcinoma. H.E., x 200

D. Lavage cytology under direct vision by the fiberscope demonstrated adenocarcinoma cells with large nucleoli and irregular distribution of chromatin substance.

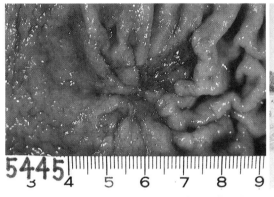

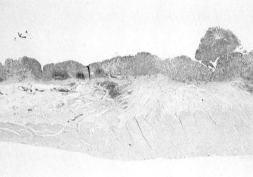

E. Gross specimen showing a 3.8 x 3.0 depressed lesion on the greater curvature of the lower body.

F. Lower power view of the histology demonstrating cancer cell infiltration limited within the mucosa and submucosa. H.E., x 1.5

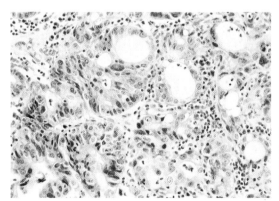

G. Histology on high power view demonstrates a moderately differentiated tubular adenocarcinoma which invades mucosal and submucosal layers. No lymph node metastases demonstrated. H.E., x 200

* Figures B, D, E and F reproduced from Kasugai, T.: Gastric lavage cytology under direct observation with the fibergastroscope. In: Murakami, T. (ed.) Early Gastric Cancer, pp.207-221, University of Tokyo Press, Tokyo, 1971.

Case 31   Flat polyp (Type I of Yamada's classification)

A 72-year-old female. *Chief complaint:* epigastric discomfort.

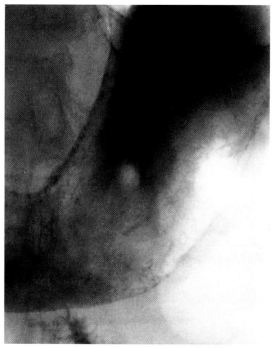

A. Barium meal study revealing a small, round defect in the lower gastric body.

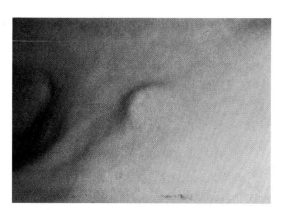 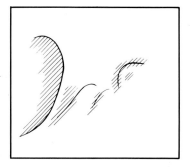

B.   Endoscopy revealing a small, flat elevation on the lesser curvature aspect of the posterior wall of the mid-body of the stomach.

Case 32   Sessile polyp (Type II of Yamada's classification)

A 54-year-old female. *Chief complaint:* epigastric fullness.

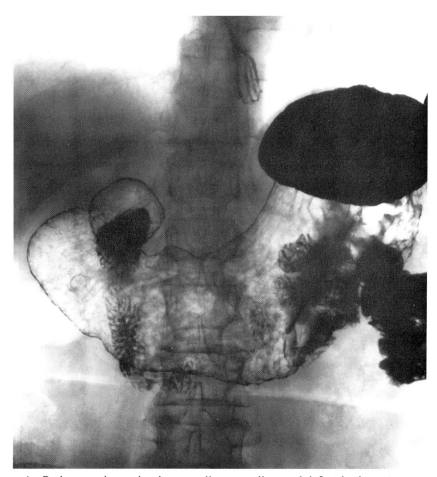

A. Barium meal examination revealing a small, round defect in the antrum.

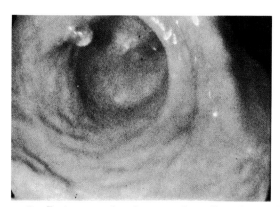 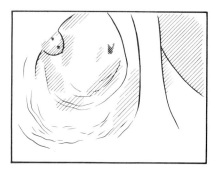

B. Endoscopy showing a small sessile polyp with redness and erosions on the anterior aspect of the antrum.

Case 33   Sessile polyp (Type II of Yamada's classification)

A 60-year-old female. *Chief complaint:* poor appetite.

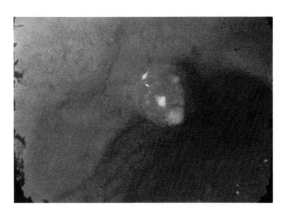 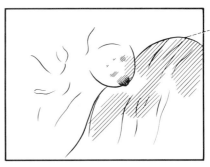

gastric
angulus

Endoscopy revealing a sessile polyp with some erosions and redness on its surface on the anterior wall of the lower body of the stomach.

Case 34 Pedunculated polyp (Type IV of Yamada's classification)

A 54-year-old male. *Chief complaint:* abdominal fullness.

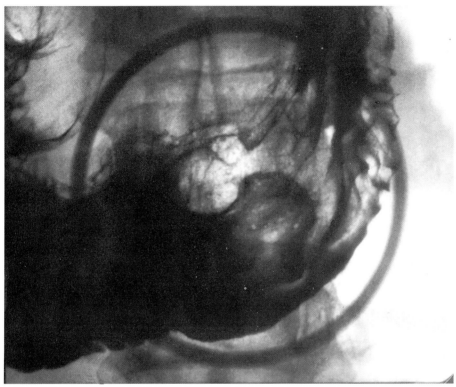

A. Barium meal examination showing a polypoid defect with a long stalk in the lower body.

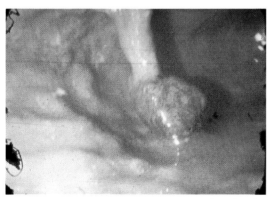
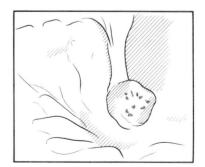

B. Endoscopy revealing a pedunculated polyp, red in color, having a long stalk and erosions on the surface, on the greater curvature aspect of the anterior wall of the lower gastric body.

Case 35   **Multiple polyps (Polyposis)**

A 64-year-old male. *Chief complaint:* anorexia.

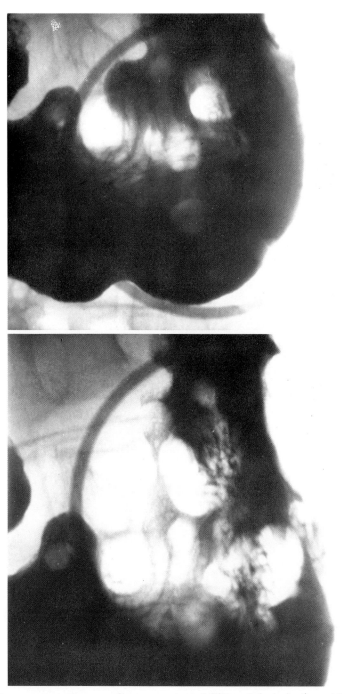

A. Barium meal studies revealing many round filling defects in the mid and lower body, and antrum.

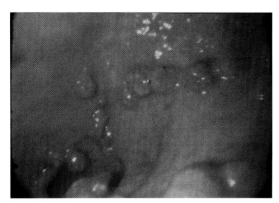 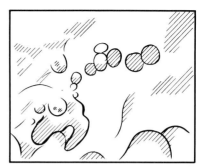

B. Endoscopy revealing multiple sessile polyps in the mid and lower body of the stomach.

Case 36   Atypical polyp of border-line malignancy, "border-line polyp"

A 49-year-old female. *Chief complaint:* epigastric pain. *Treatment:* followed up six times by endoscopy with biopsy in two years and partial gastrectomy.

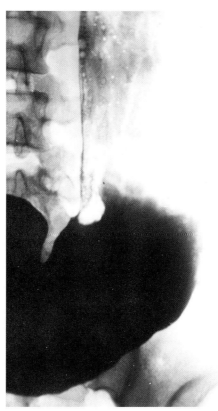

A. A barium meal examination revealing an oval filling defect on the lesser curvature aspect of the stomach.

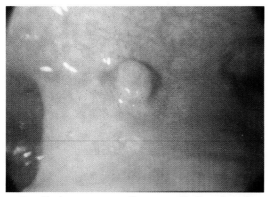
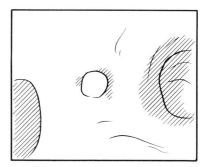

B. Endoscopy revealing a small, flat elevation covered with smooth mucosa, pale in color, on the lesser curvature of the lower gastric body.

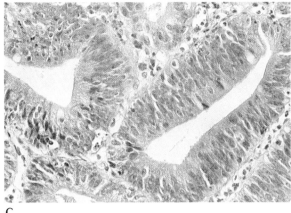

C

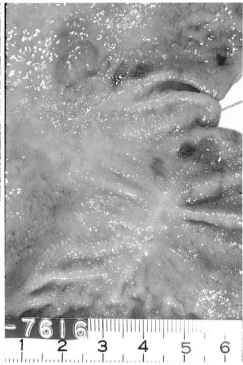

C. Biopsy demonstrates atypical epithelium—border-
line malignancy. H.E., x 200

D. Surgically resected specimen shows a small flat
elevation, 1.2 x 0.8 x 0.4 cm in size, on the anterior
aspect of the lesser curvature of the lower gastric
body, and a linear ulcer scar with converging folds on
the posterior wall.

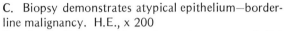

D

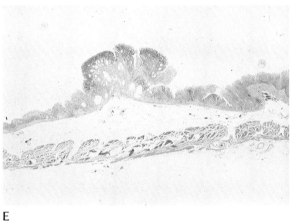

E

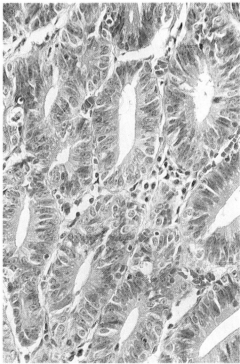

E. Low power histology of the specimen shows a
small polypoid lesion of the mucosa. H.E., x 1.5

F. Histology of the specimen demonstrates fairly advanced atypia in cellular and structural pattern with
numerous mitoses and may be regarded as "carcinoma in situ" in nature; Atypical polyp of border-line
malignancy, "border-line polyp". H.E., x 200

F

Case 37 **Leiomyoma**

A 38-year-old female. *Chief complaint:* asymptomatic, but occasional constipation. *Treatment:* follow-up by endoscopy with biopsy and upper GI radiography every year in the past eight years.

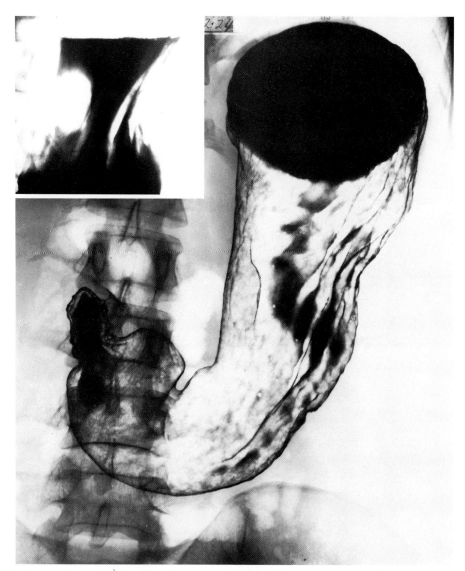

A. Barium meal examination revealing an oval filling defect with a smooth outline, 3.5 x 2.3 cm in diameter, on the posterior wall of the mid-body of the stomach.

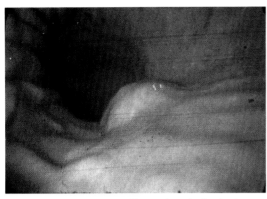 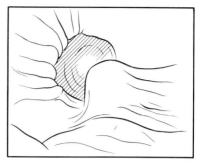

B. Endoscopy revealing a hemispherical tumor covered with normal gastric mucosa accompanied by bridging folds on the posterior wall of the mid-body. Biopsy showed chronic gastritis without evidence of malignancy.

Case 38   **Leiomyoma**

A 74-year-old female. *Chief complaint:* asymptomatic. She died of cerebral apoplexy one year and nine months after the first examination.

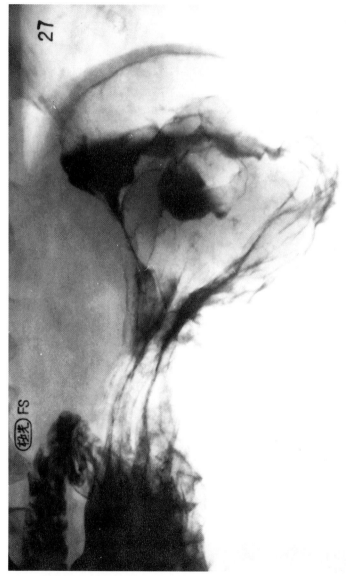

A. Barium meal examination revealing a round tumorous mass with a huge ulceration on the posterior aspect of the gastric fornix.

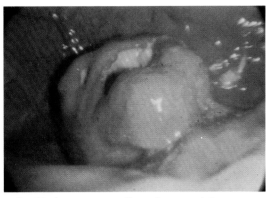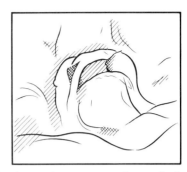

B. Endoscopy revealing a huge nodular tumor with a large, deep crater and a small ulcer on the posterior aspect of the fornix.

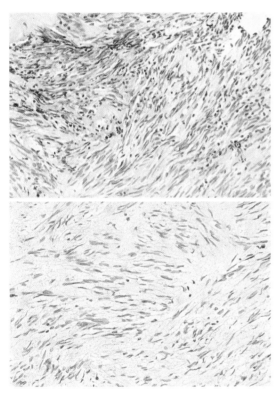

C. Biopsy of the ulcer floor demonstrates myogenic tumor cells. H.E., x 200

D. Histology demonstrates leiomyoma tissue. H.E., x 200

Case 39 **Aberrant pancreas**

A 52-year-old male. *Chief complaint:* epigastric pain. *Treatment:* partial gastrectomy was performed for gastric cancer of the gastric body.

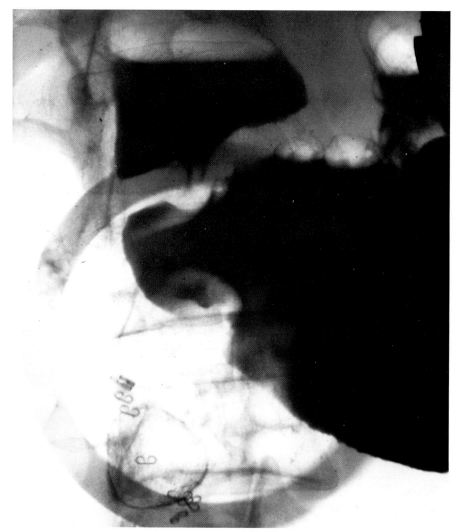

A. Barium meal examination revealing a semicircular filling defect with a central depression on the greater curvature of the antrum.

115

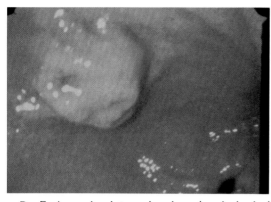 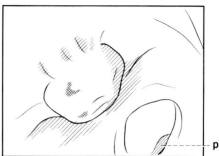 pylorus

B. Endoscopic picture showing a hemispherical tumor with bridging folds and a central depression on the anterior aspect of the greater curvature of the antrum.

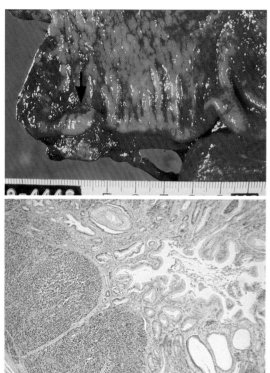

C. Surgically resected specimen showing a hemispherical elevation with a central depression (arrow), 1.0 x 1.0 cm in size, on the greater curvature of the antrum.

D. Histology of the specimen demonstrating heterotopic pancreatic tissues consisting of acinar tissue with pancreatic ductules. H.E., x 40

Case 40   Aberrant pancreas

A 40-year-old female. *Chief complaint:* asymptomatic, detected on gastric mass survey. *Treatment:* partial gastrectomy.

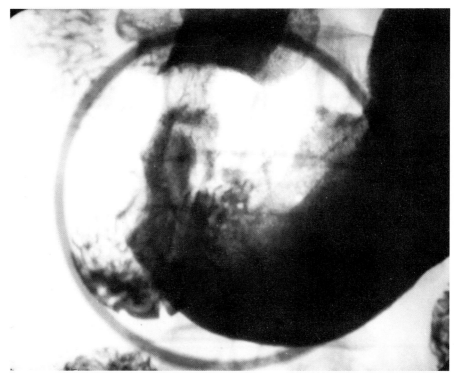

A. Barium meal study showing a smooth, flat semicircular defect on the greater curvature of the antrum.

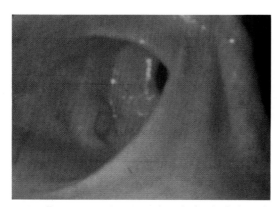
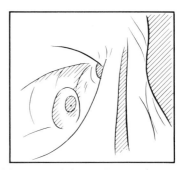

B. Endoscopy showing a hemispherical elevation with a central depression on the greater curvature of the antrum.

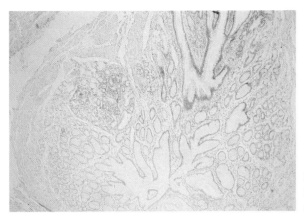

C. Histology of the specimen demonstrating heterotopic pancreatic ducts, associated with acinar tissue. H.E., x 200

Case 41   Syphilis of the stomach

A 29-year-old female. *Chief complaints:* severe epigastric pain and vomiting. Serology for syphilis was positive. *Treatment:* partial gastrectomy.

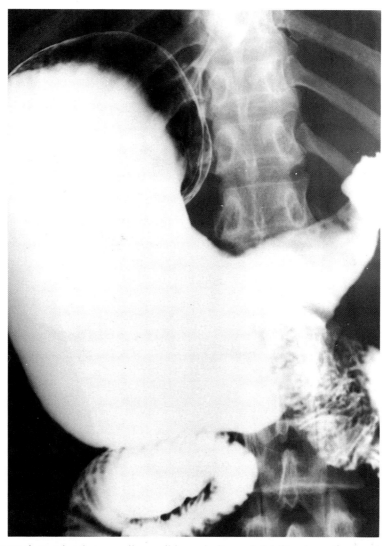

A. Barium meal examination revealing wall irregularity and rigidity above the angulus down to the antrum.

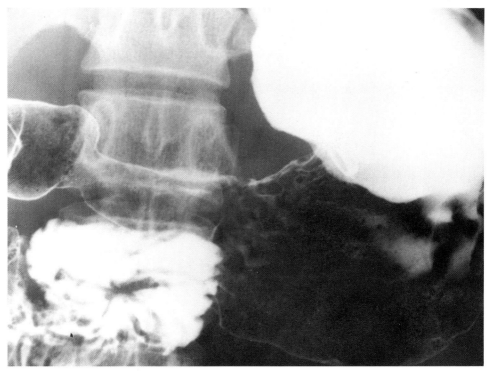

B. Double contrast radiogram revealing mucosal destruction and barium flecks in the lower body and antrum.

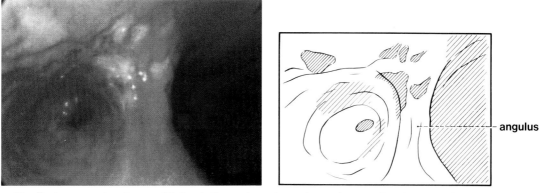

C. Endoscopy showing multiple shallow ulcers just above the angulus down to the antrum, which are round or irregular in shape with a dirty yellowish coat. The edges are smooth and sharp and the surrounding areas are dull reddish orange. The ulcers are creeping and spreading distally.

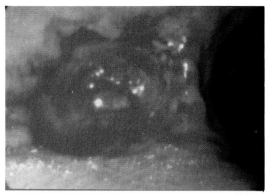
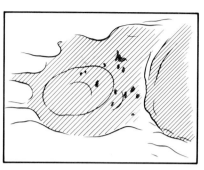

D. Endoscopy taken 20 days later, showing mucosal destruction just above the angulus all the way down to the antrum, which was covered with a dull, smooth slime, and during this period it had changed to a reddish flesh color with bleeding.

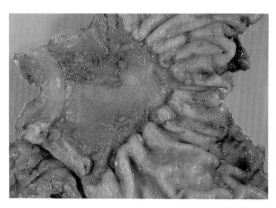

E. Surgically resected specimen showing destruction of the mucosa as a huge ulcer from lower body to all of the distal antrum with converging folds, the ends of which are smoothly round.

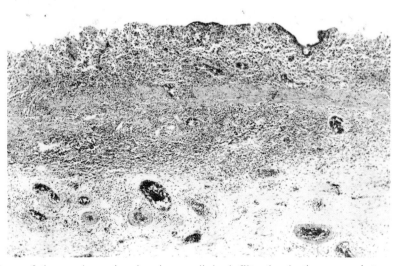

F. Histology of the specimen showing dense cellular infiltration in the mucosal stroma and the upper layer of the submucosa. Vascular engorgement and perivascular infiltration present. H.E., x 40

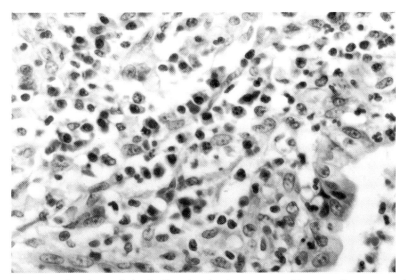

G. High power view showing cellular infiltration in the mucosa. Plasma cells are conspicuous in this field. Glandular epithelium is on the right. H.E., x 400

Case 42   Tuberculosis of the stomach*

A 35-year-old female. *Chief complaint:* nausea. Tuberculous reaction was positive and chest X-ray film revealed no active disease and no calcification. *Treatment:* healed with chemotherapy.

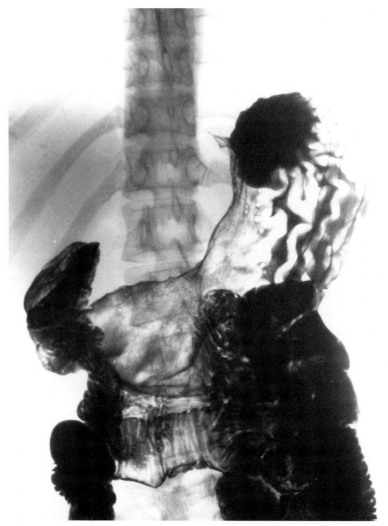

A. Barium meal examination revealing many tiny niches on the lesser curvature of the lower body and antrum.

* From Ito, Y., Kobayashi, S., and Kasugai, T.: A case of gastric tuberculosis. Gastroenterol. Endosc. 17: 426-431, 1975.

123

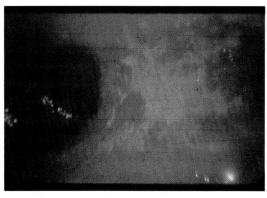
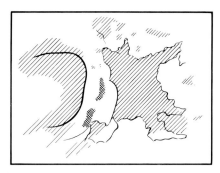

B. Endoscopy showing many irregularly shaped shallow ulcers varying in size on the lesser curvature of the lower body of the stomach.

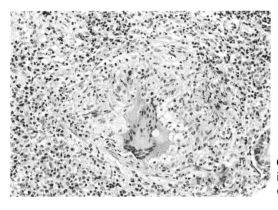

C. Biopsy demonstrating tubercles consisting of giant cells of Langhans type and epithelioid cells. H.E., x 200

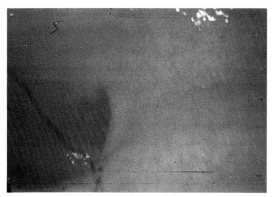
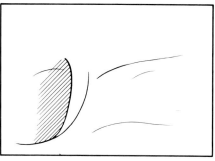

D. Endoscopy after 20 weeks of chemotherapy with streptomycin, para-aminosalicylic acid (PAS) and isonicotine hydrazine (INH) revealing no lesion.

Case 43   Gastric carcinoid

A 32-year-old male. *Chief complaint:* epigastric fullness. *Laboratory data:* blood serotonin, 12.7 mg/dl; urine 5-HIAA, 0.7–3.0 mg/24 hr; urine 17 KS, 14.1 mg/24 hr; urine 17-OHCS, 7.4 mg/24 hr; GTT (50g), diabetic pattern; urinary sugar (−). *Treatment:* partial gastrectomy.

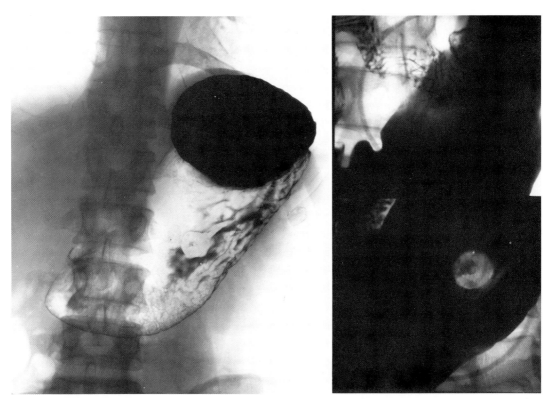

A. Barium meal examination revealing a round filling defect, 2.0 x 2.0 cm in diameter, with a central ulceration with a bridging fold, on the posterior wall of the lower body.

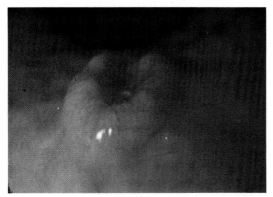
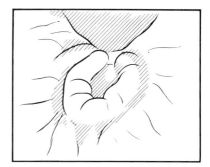

B. Endoscopy revealing a tumor with a large central depression, with bridging folds on the posterior wall of the lower body.

125

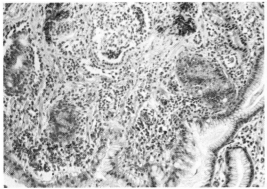

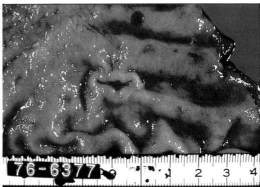

C. Biopsy strongly suggests carcinoid tumor. H.E., x 100

D. Surgically resected specimen showing a flat tumor, 1.2 x 1.8 cm in size, with a deep, central depression on the posterior wall of the lower body.

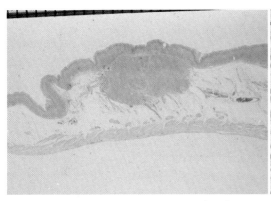

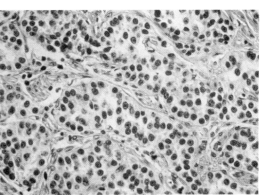

E. Histology of low power view showing a lesion mainly in the submucosal layer, with the mucosal layer partially involved.

F. Histology demonstrating carcinoid tumor. H.E., x 200

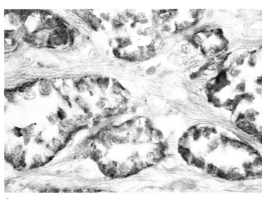

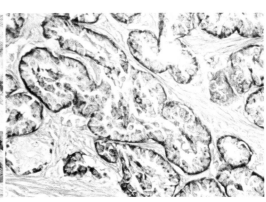

G

H

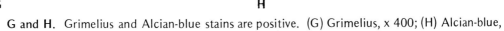

G and H. Grimelius and Alcian-blue stains are positive. (G) Grimelius, x 400; (H) Alcian-blue, x 200

Case 44   **Leiomyosarcoma**

A 35-year-old female. *Chief complaints:* epigastric pain and anemia. *Treatment:* partial gastrectomy.

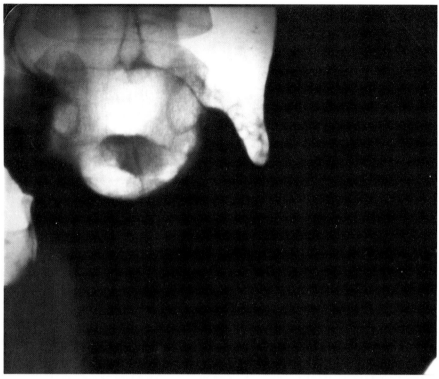

A. Barium meal study revealing a huge, round filling defect with a central ulceration on the lesser curvature aspect of the antrum.

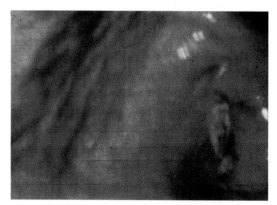 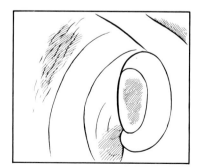

B. Endoscopy revealing a huge ulcer with a thick, smooth wall covered with normal-appearing mucosa on the lesser curvature aspect of the antrum.

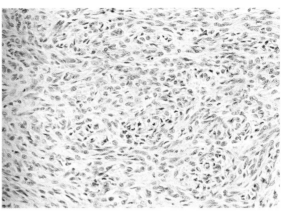

D

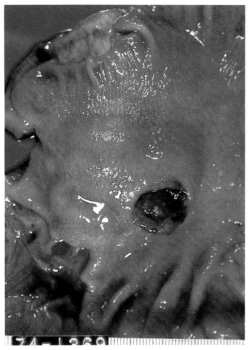

C

C. Surgically resected specimen showing an irregularly shaped hemispherical tumor covered with normal-
appearing mucosa, with a deep central ulceration accompanied by some bridging folds in the antrum.
D. Histology of the specimen demonstrating leiomyosarcoma of low grade malignancy. H.E., x 200

Case 45   Leiomyosarcoma

A 45-year-old male. *Chief complaints:* anorexia and weight loss. *Treatment:* proximal gastrectomy.

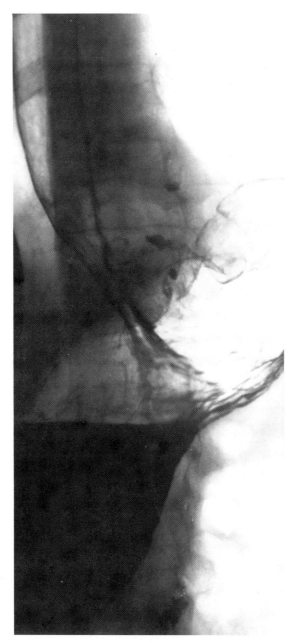

A. Barium meal examination revealing an irregularly shaped filling defect in the cardia and fornix.

129

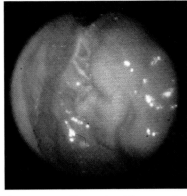
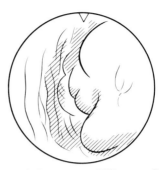

B. Endoscopy performed with a gastrointestinal fiberscope GIF type P2 showing a huge nodular tumor with a central ulcer in the fornix.

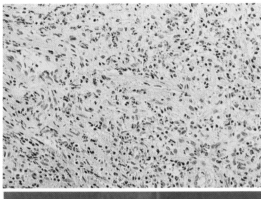

C. Biopsy demonstrates myxomatous tissues. Alcian-blue, x 200

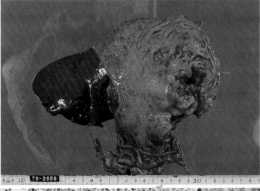

D. Gross specimen showing a huge nodular tumor with a deep central crater in the fornix near the cardia.

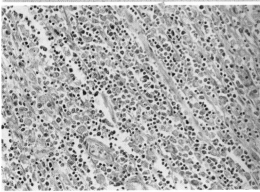

E. Histology of the specimen demonstrating leiomyosarcoma tissues. H.E., x 200

Case 46   Malignant lymphoma

A 66-year-old female. *Chief complaint:* heaviness in the epigastrium. *Treatment:* partial gastrectomy after irradiation.

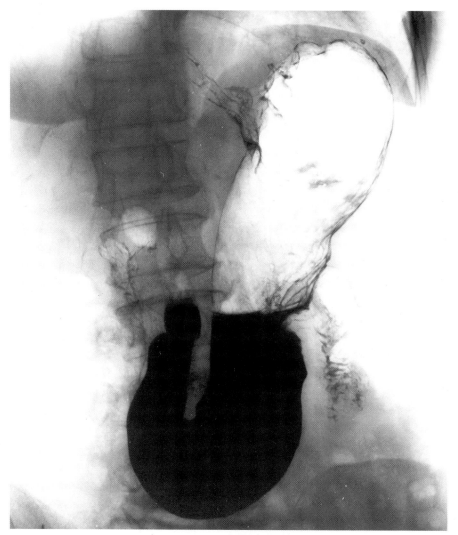

A. X-ray examination revealing an irregular filling defect in the cardiac area.

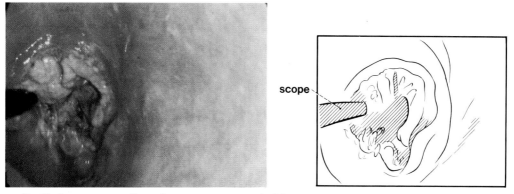

B. Endoscopy revealing a huge crater covered with a thick creamy and bloody coat surrounded by a bright crater wall in the cardiac area.

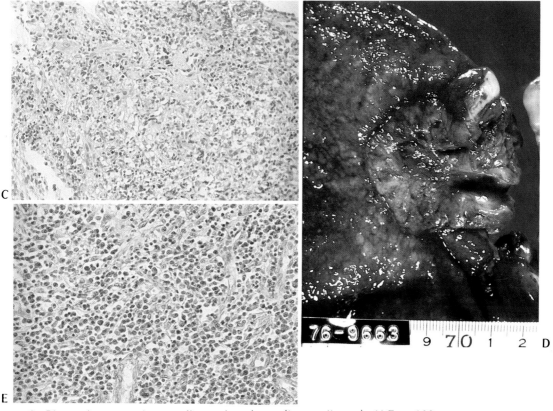

C. Biopsy demonstrating a malignant lymphoma (large cell type). H.E., x 200
D. Surgically resected specimen showing a huge crater, 5.0 x 4.0 cm in size, in the gastric cardia.
E. Histology of the specimen demonstrating a malignant lymphoma (large cell type) after irradiation. H.E., x 200

Case 47   Malignant lymphoma

A 62-year-old male. *Chief complaint:* epigastric pain in the fasting period. *Treatment:* partial gastrectomy.

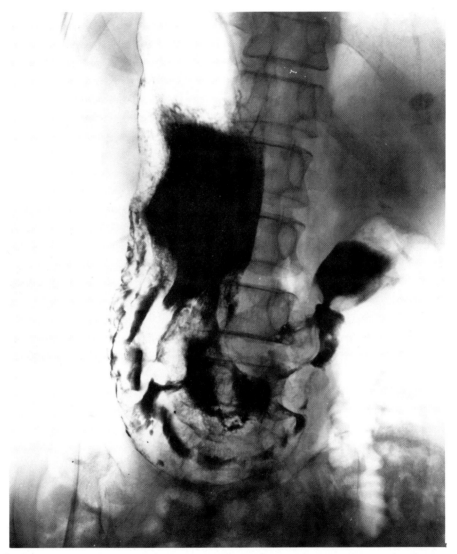

A. Barium meal study taken with patient in the prone position revealing coarse giant folds in the mid and lower body and filling defect in the lower body and antrum, mainly on the anterior aspect.

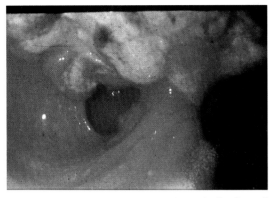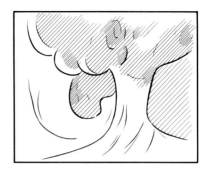

B. Endoscopy revealing an irregularly shaped huge ulcer covered with a thick, creamy, bloody and dirty coat on the anterior wall of the lower body and antrum.

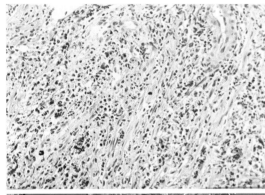

C. Biopsy demonstrating a malignant lymphoma (large cell type). H.E., x 200

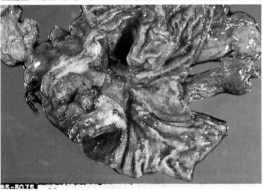

D. Surgically resected specimen showing a huge crater in the lower body and antrum.

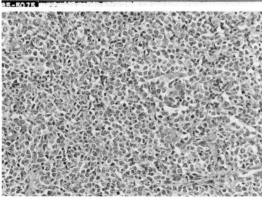

E. Histology of the specimen demonstrating a malignant lymphoma (large cell type). H.E., x 200

Case 48   Malignant lymphoma

A 21-year-old male. *Chief complaint:* epigastric pain. *Treatment:* partial gastrectomy.

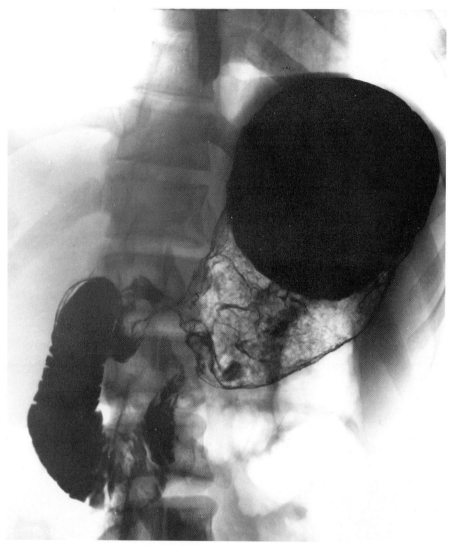

A. Barium meal study revealing a marked filling defect in the antrum with tumorous folds in the lower body.

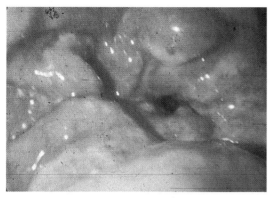
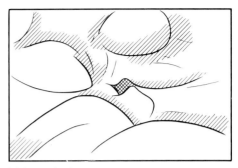

B. Endoscopy showing many nodular folds which made the antrum very narrow.

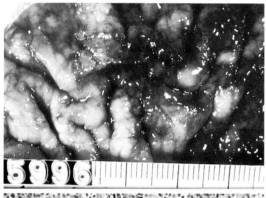

C. Surgically resected specimen showing numerous, nodular giant folds in the antrum.

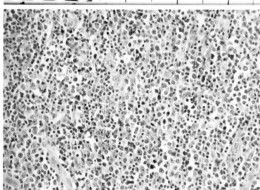

D. Histology of the specimen demonstrating a malignant lymphoma (large cell type). H.E., x 200

Case 49 Gastric bezoar

A 63-year-old male. *Chief complaint:* asymptomatic. He was picked up on a gastric mass survey. *Treatment:* removal of the bezoar by gastrotomy.

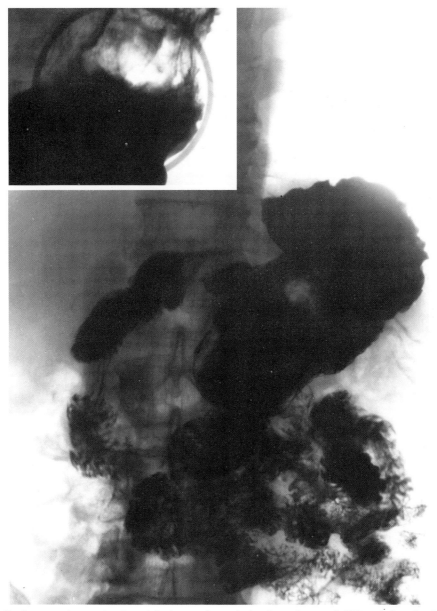

A. Barium meal examination showing an irregularly shaped, round filling defect in the body which could be easily moved.

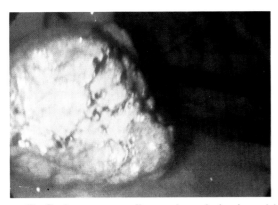 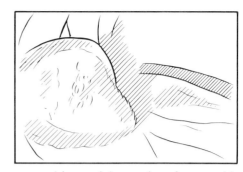

B. Endoscopy revealing an irregularly shaped large mass with a nodular rough surface, grayish red brown in color which was moved by changing the patient's position.

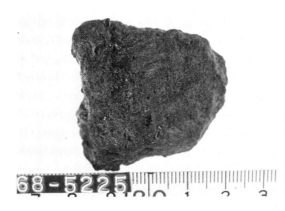

C. Removed specimen. Iniobezoar with a size of 5 x 4 x 3 cm, weighing 22.5 g and having a color of red brown, shows nodularly rough surface with partially gray-white adherent material like mold and cork-like elastic softness.

Case 50 Gastric varix

An 18-year-old female. *Chief complaint:* hematemesis.

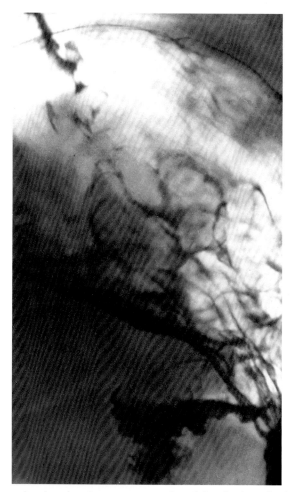

A. Barium meal examination showing many netted nodular shadows in the cardia and fornix.

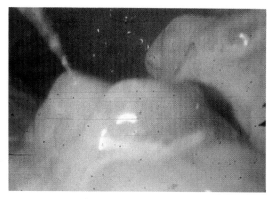
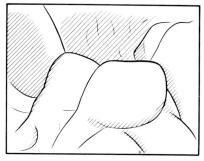

B. Endoscopy revealing multiple smooth, nodular elevations in the cardiac area.

Case 51 Gastric varix

A 62-year-old female. *Chief complaint:* epigastric fullness.

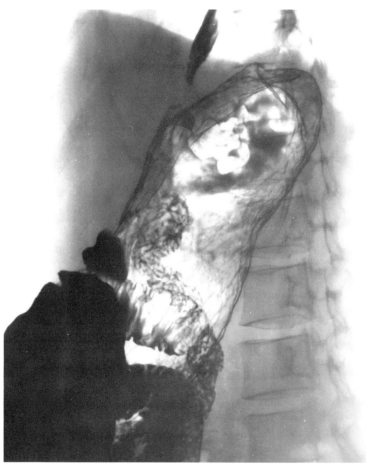

A. Barium meal examination showing a giant fold-like defect in the cardia and fornix.

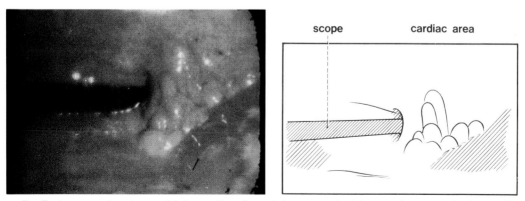

B. Endoscopy showing multiple small, soft nodules covered with smooth mucosa in the cardia and fornix.

Case 52 Gastric diverticulum

A 47-year-old male. *Chief complaint:* asymptomatic. He was picked up on a gastric mass survey.

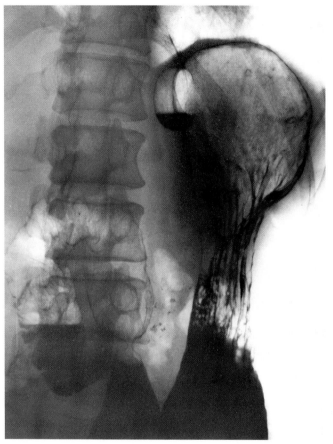

A. Barium meal study revealing an oval pouch in the cardiac area.

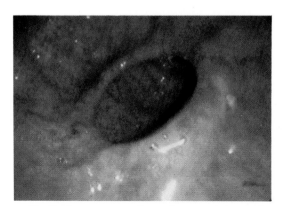
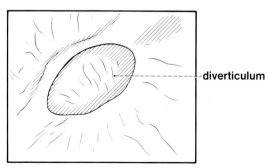

B. Endoscopy revealing a huge oval depression, the floor of which is covered with normal gastric mucosa, on the posterior wall of the cardiac area.

Case 53 Gastric diverticulum

A 27-year-old male. *Chief complaint:* epigastric fullness.

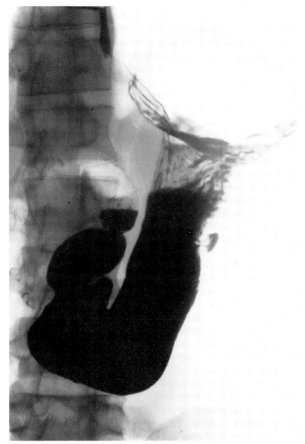

A. Barium meal examination showing a small protruded shadow on the greater curvature of the mid-body.

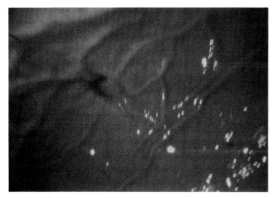
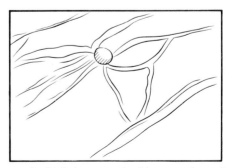

B. Endoscopy showing an oval depression, the floor of which is covered with normal gastric mucosa, on the greater curvature of the mid-body. The gastric folds merge smoothly into the depression.

4

Endoscopy of the Duodenum

TATSUZO KASUGAI, M.D.

Indications

Duodenoscopy is indicated to confirm the presence of a duodenal ulcer or its scar in all patients in whom a barium meal examination is consistent with such a lesion. It is especially indicated prior to surgical treatment for duodenal ulcer, and for a healing ulcer which is hardly visualized on X-ray examination.

Observation and biopsy of the papilla of Vater are important in endoscopy of the second portion of the duodenum.

Furthermore, duodenoscopy with or without biopsy is performed to evaluate the existence and nature — benign or malignant — of lesions in the duodenum.

Instruments

Both forward- and side-viewing instruments are used for duodenoscopy. The forward-viewing duodenoscope is more convenient for observation of the duodenal bulb: however, side-views as JF type B4 (Fig. 4-1) or Fujinon QB (Fig. 4-2) are preferable for observation, biopsy and cannulation of the papilla of Vater.

Premedication

Duodenoscopy requires the same preparation of patients as other endoscopic procedures of the upper gastrointestinal tract.

Technique

Duodenoscopy is performed with the patient in the left lateral decubitus position, as for other endoscopic procedures of the upper gastrointestinal tract. The pyloric ring is easily passed under direct vision with a forward-viewing endoscope.

On the other hand, a special technique is required to pass the pylorus with a side-viewing duodenoscope because the pylorus is passed blindly.

The tip of the side-viewing duodenoscope is advanced as close to the pylorus as possible and the pylorus is brought into the center of the visual field en face. Next, the tip is deflected upward to visualize the lesser curvature of the antrum, and the scope is slowly pushed forward simultaneously with air insufflation. The tip enters easily into the duodenal bulb and is advanced by clockwise rotation of the scope with its up-angle, into the entrance of the second portion of the duodenum beyond the superior duodenal angle.

The scope is then advanced under direct vision with its counterclockwise rotation until the longitudinal fold of the papilla of Vater comes into view. The papilla of

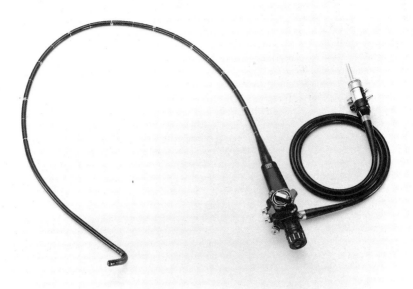

Fig. 4-1 Olympus duodenofiberscope J F type B4 (side-viewing).

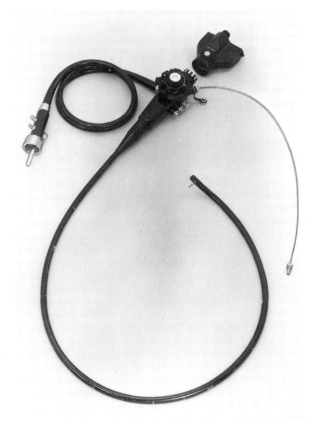

Fig. 4-2 Fujinon duodenofiberscope FD-QB (side-viewing).

Vater, which is located at the distal end of the longitudinal fold, is visualized by advancing the scope further.

In contrast to this, the tip of the scope is advanced to visualize the papilla of Vater beyond the superior duodenal angle by withdrawing the scope during clockwise rotation of the scope with the up-angle of the tip with the patient in the prone position, because unwinding the loop of the scope in the stomach presses the tip forward.

In cases where the papilla of Vater is not detected upon introduction of the duodenoscope into the proximal part of the second portion of the duodenum, it is advisable to advance the instrument to the junction of the second and third portions of the duodenum. The endoscope is then withdrawn slowly with constant inspection of the inner aspect of the duodenal wall until the papilla comes into view. Its appearance is indicated by the frenulum of the papilla of Vater. The minor papilla is usually found about 2 cm above and a little to the right side in the visual field. A schema of the papilla of Vater is shown in Figure 4-3.

The duodenoscope can be advanced easily to the duodenojejunal junction when examination of the entire duodenum is clinically indicated.

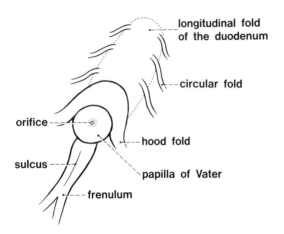

Fig. 4-3 Schematic drawing of the papilla of Vater.

Results

Correlation between X-ray and endoscopic findings of duodenal ulcer disease is shown in Table 4-1. Duodenal ulcer scars, pouches or linear ulcers were commonly observed in the deformed duodenal bulb demonstrated by a barium meal study, however, round or irregularly shaped open ulcers were also occasionally found in such cases.

Small elevations which are usually benign are occasionally observed in the duodenal bulb. If a malignant lesion is confirmed by biopsy, it will usually be invasion from a malignant lesion of another organ, mainly the biliary system.

Acute or chronic inflammation of the papilla of Vater called papillitis is occasionally observed in patients with biliary or pancreatic diseases. Primary carcinoma of the papilla of Vater as well as papillary invasion from carcinoma of the head of the pancreas are detected endoscopy and biopsy.

Table 4-1 Correlation between X-ray and endoscopic findings of duodenal ulcer diseases.

Endoscopic findings \ X-ray findings	Niche deformity converging folds	Niche deformity	Niche converging folds	Niche	Niches	Deformity	Deformity converging folds	Converging folds	Normal	Total
Ulcer										
Round		41	2	20	1	15	4		3	86
Irregular	1	16		6		11			2	36
Linear		17		5		13	1	1		37
Pepper and salt		4				3	1		1	9
Scar										
Common type	2	20		6		38	15	2	12	95
Linear		3				6	1			10
Pouch		11		1		24	6			42
Marked deformity		7		2		7				16
Duodenitis						1				1
Normal		1		2						3
Total	3	120	2	42	1	118	28	3	18	335

Including 36 cases of kissing ulcers and the scar, and 6 of multiple ulcers.

REFERENCES

1) Belber, J.P.: Duodenal bulb visualization with the Hirchowitz gastroduodenal fiberscope and the Hirschowitz gastroduodenal fiberscope with deflecting tip: A comparative study. Gastrointest. Endosc. 17: 34-35, 1970.

2) Hirschowitz, B.I., Balint, J.A., and Fulton, W.F.: Gastroduodenal endoscopy with the fiberscope: An analysis of 500 cases. Surg. Clin. N. Amer. 42: 1081-1090, 1962.

3) Kasugai, T., Kuno, N., Aoki, I., Kizu, M., and Kobayashi, S.: Fiberduodenoscopy: Analysis of 353 examinations. Gastrointest. Endosc. 18: 9-16, 1971.

Case 1 Normal duodenal bulb

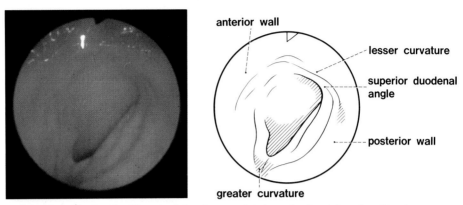

A. Normal duodenal bulb of a 70-year-old male complaining of epigastric pain. Duodenoscopy was performed with a duodenofiberscope JF type B4.

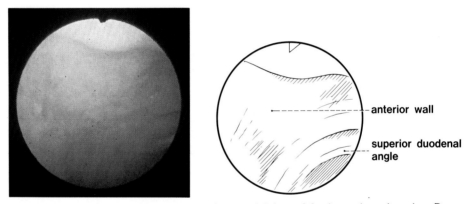

B. Normal duodenal bulb of a 44-year-old male complaining of fasting epigastric pain. Duodenoscopy was performed with a duodenofiberscope JF type B4.

Case 2   Duodenal ulcer

A 39-year-old male. *Chief complaint:* fasting epigastric pain.

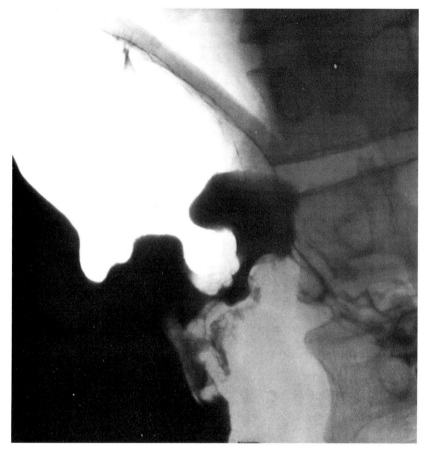

A. Barium meal study taken with the patient in the prone position revealing a markedly deformed bulb with a niche.

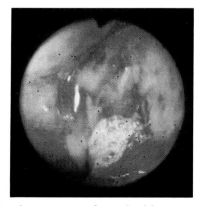 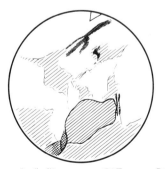

B. Duodenoscopy performed with a gastrointestinal fiberscope GIF type P2 reveals a large ulcer with a white covering in the lesser curvature of the deformed duodenal bulb.

Case 3   Duodenal ulcer

A 38-year-old male. *Chief complaint:* fasting epigastric pain.

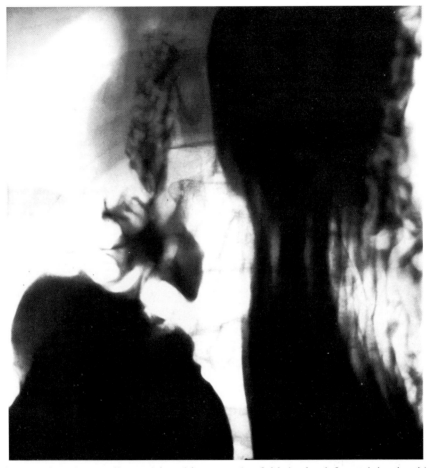

A. Barium meal study revealing a niche with converging folds in the deformed duodenal bulb.

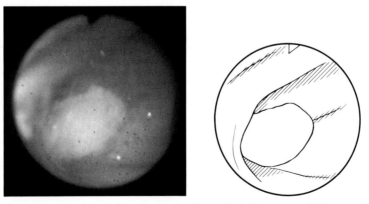

B. Duodenoscopy performed with a gastrointestinal fiberscope GIF type P2 reveals a large, round ulcer with a white coating on the anterior wall of the duodenal bulb.

Case 4   Kissing duodenal ulcers

A 41-year-old male. *Chief complaint:* epigastric pain.

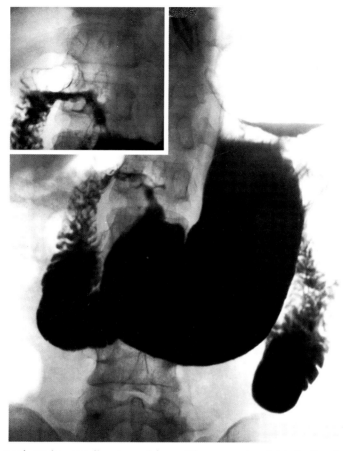

A. Barium meal study revealing two niches with converging folds in the deformed duodenal bulb.

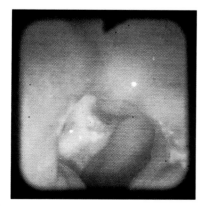
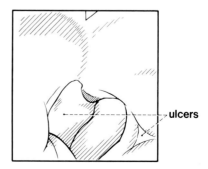

B. Duodenoscopy performed with a duodenofiberscope JF type B3 reveals two irregularly shaped ulcers, a large one on the anterior wall and a small one on the posterior wall respectively.

Case 5   Linear duodenal ulcer

A 45-year-old female. *Chief complaints:* epigastric pain and nausea.

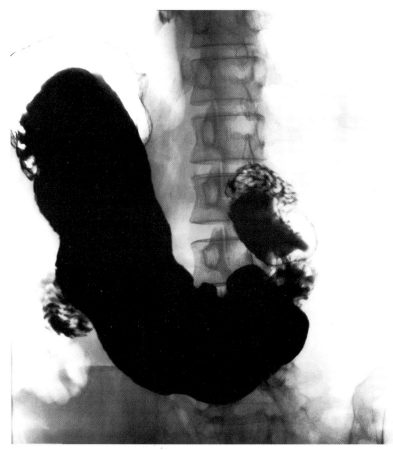

A. Barium meal study taken with the patient in the prone position revealing a deformed duodenal bulb.

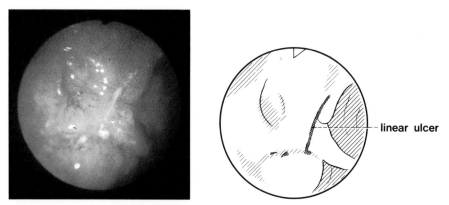

B. Duodenoscopy performed with a duodenofiberscope JF type B3 shows an irregularly shaped linear ulcer with some converging folds on the anterior wall of the deformed bulb.

Case 6 Duodenal ulcer scar

A 45-year-old male. *Chief complaints:* heartburn and epigastric discomfort.

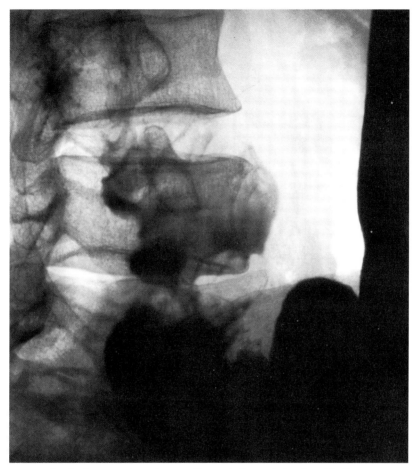

A. Barium meal study revealing a deformed duodenal bulb.

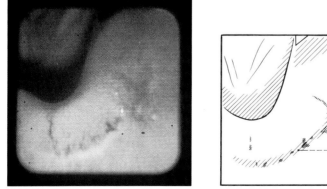

linear ulcer scar

B. Duodenoscopy performed with a duodenofiberscope JF type B3 shows a linear ulcer scar on the posterior wall of the duodenal bulb.

Case 7 **Duodenal ulcer scar with pouches**

A 52-year-old male. *Chief complaint:* asymptomatic.

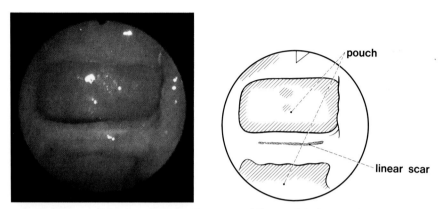

Duodenoscopy performed with a duodenofiberscope JF type B3 shows a linear ulcer scar with pouches on the anterior wall of the deformed duodenal bulb.

Case 8 Duodenal diverticulum

A 65-year-old male. *Chief complaint:* asymptomatic.

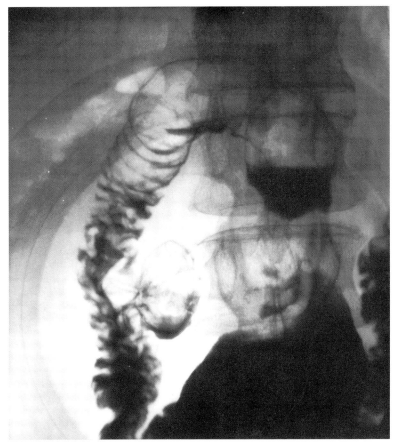

A. Barium meal examination revealing a diverticulum on the inner wall of the second portion of the duodenum.

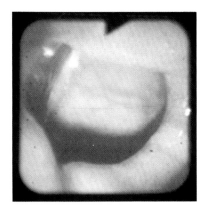
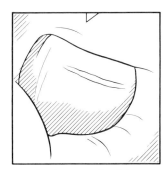

B. Duodenoscopy showing a large diverticulum on the inner wall of the second portion of the duodenum.

Case 9   Duodenal carcinoma

A 55-year-old male. *Chief complaint:* right abdominal pain. *Treatment:* pancreato-duodenectomy.

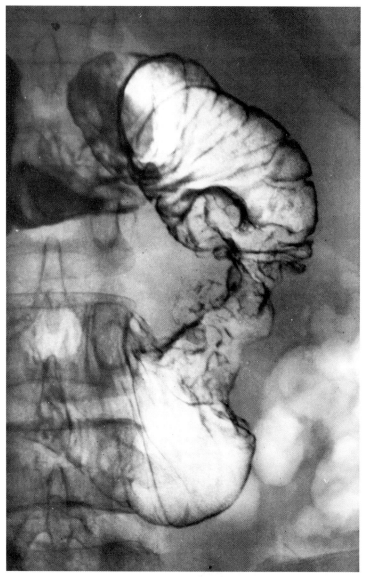

A. Hypotonic duodenogram revealing an apple core-like defect in the distal part of the second portion of the duodenum.

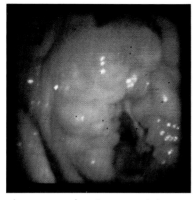 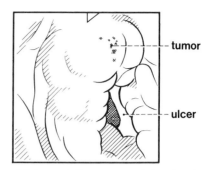

B. Duodenoscopy showing a nodular tumor, which partially narrowed the duodenal cavity, with an irregular ulceration in the distal part of the second portion of the duodenum.

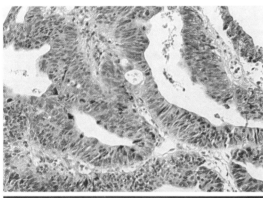

C. Biopsy demonstrating a papillo-tubular adenocarcinoma. H.E., x 200

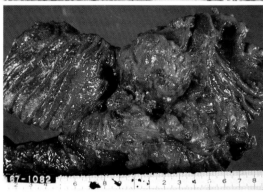

D. Surgically resected specimen showing a tumor, 8.0 x 7.5 cm in size, in the second portion of the duodenum.

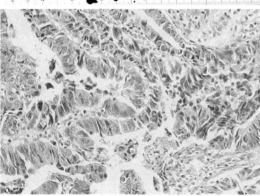

E. Histology of the specimen demonstrating a well-differentiated papillary adenocarcinoma. H.E., x 200

Case 10   Normal papilla of Vater

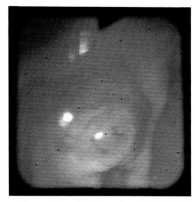 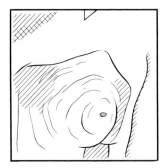

A. Normal papilla of Vater, hemispherical type, with a round orifice. Duodenoscopy of a 32-year-old male complaining of right upper quadrant pain.

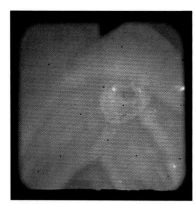 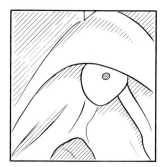

B. Normal papilla of Vater, hemispherical type, with a round orifice. Duodenoscopy of a 50-year-old female complaining of weight loss.

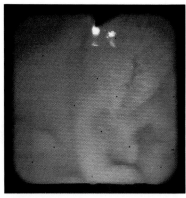 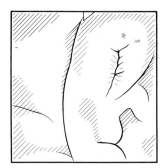

C. Normal papilla of Vater, hemiellipsoid type, with an elongated orifice. Duodenoscopy of a 36-year-old female complaining of poor appetite.

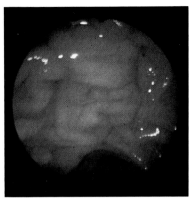 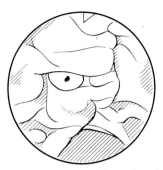

D. Normal papilla of Vater, hemispherical type, with a slit-like orifice. Duodenoscopy of a 63-year-old male complaining of fasting epigastric pain.

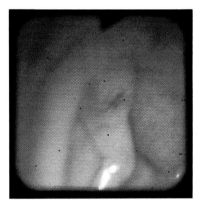 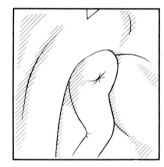

E. Normal papilla of Vater, flat type with a puckered orifice. Duodenoscopy of a 41-year-old male complaining of abdominal fullness.

Case 11   Normal papilla of Vater with separate orifices

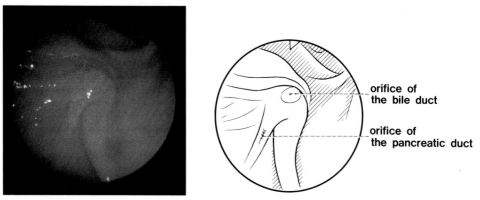

A. Normal papilla of Vater with two separate orifices. Duodenoscopy of a 45-year-old female complaining of poor appetite.

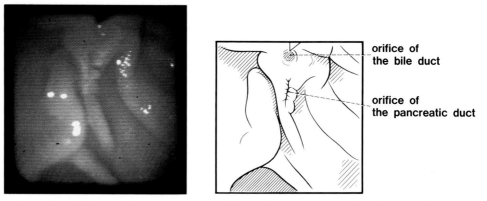

B. Normal papilla of Vater with two separate orifices. Duodenoscopy of a 48-year-old male complaining of epigastric pain.

Case 12 Papillitis

A 68-year-old male with a history of diabetes mellitus and chronic pancreatitis. *Chief complaints:* anorexia and nausea.

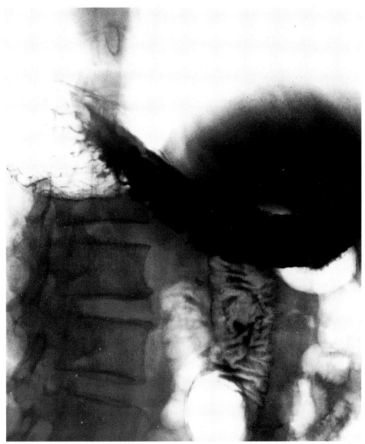

A. Hypotonic duodenogram showing a swelling of the papilla of Vater.

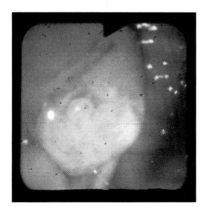 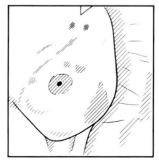

B. Duodenoscopy showing a swelling of the papilla of Vater with edema and erosions on its surface.

Case 13 Papillitis

A 60-year-old male with a history of choledocholithiasis. *Chief complaints:* jaundice and right upper quadrant pain.

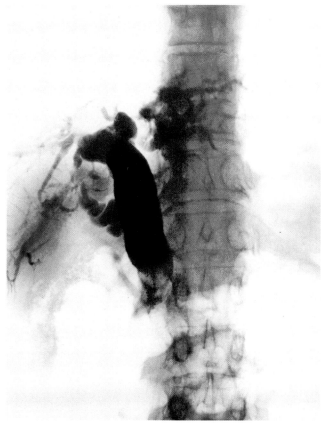

A. Endoscopic retrograde cholangiogram (ERC) revealing some radiolucencies probably due to stones in the distal portion of the markedly dilated common bile duct.

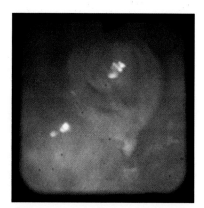 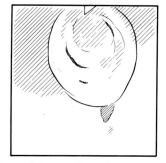

B. Duodenoscopy revealing a prominent swelling of the papilla of Vater which shows redness and edema.

Case 14   Cancer of the papilla of Vater

A 61-year-old female. *Chief complaints:* abdominal pain and fever. *Treatment:* pancreatoduodenectomy.

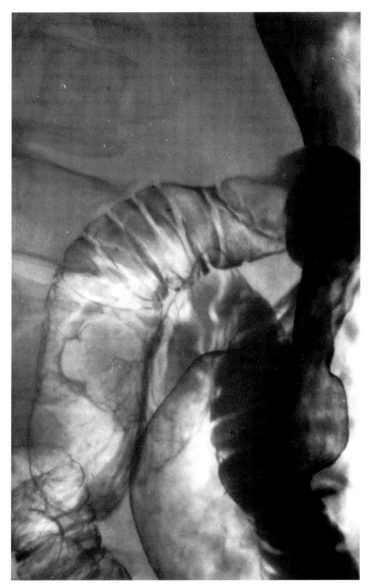

A.   Hypotonic duodenogram showing an irregularly shaped, large tumor at the area of the papilla of Vater.

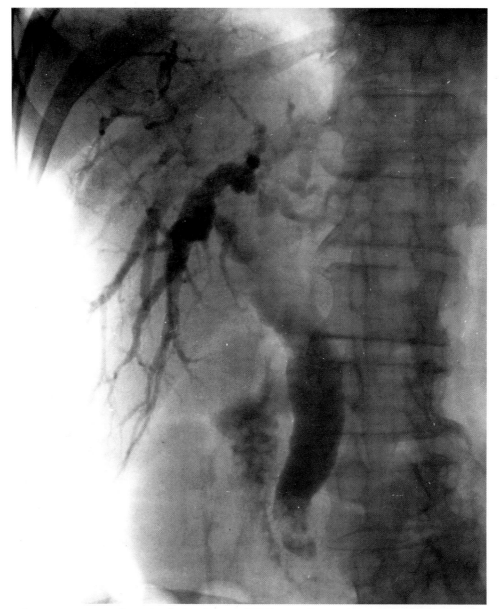

B. Percutaneous transhepatic cholangiogram (PTC) revealing an irregularly shaped elevation, 3.0 cm in size, with a granular surface at the distal part of the markedly dilated common bile duct.

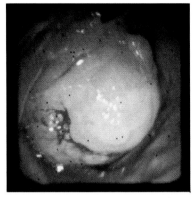
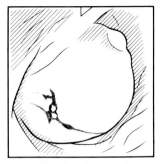

C. Duodenoscopy revealing a large spherical tumor with bleeding at the area of the papilla of Vater.

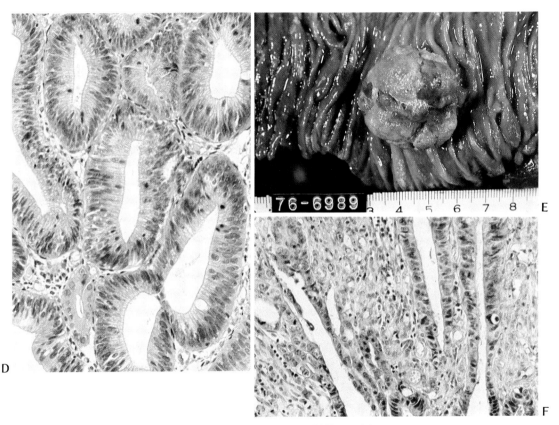

D. Biopsy demonstrating a papillary adenocarcinoma. H.E., x 200
E. Surgically resected specimen showing a papillary tumor, 4.0 x 3.5 x 2.0 cm in size, at the area of the papilla of Vater.
F. Histology of the specimen demonstrating a well-differentiated papillotubular adenocarcinoma of the papilla of Vater. H.E., x 200

Case 15 Cancer of the papilla of Vater due to invasion from cancer of the pancreatic head

A 59-year-old male. *Chief complaint:* jaundice. *Treatment:* cholecystoduodenostomy.

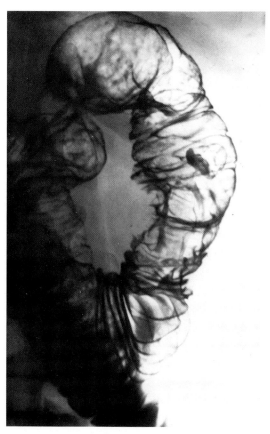

A. Hypotonic duodenogram revealing a filling defect with spiculations at the area of the papilla of Vater on the inner margin of the second portion of the duodenum.

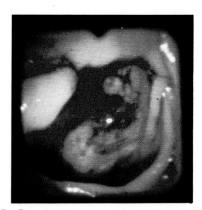 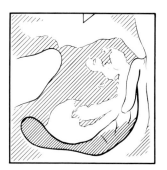

B. Duodenoscopy showing a tumorous papilla of Vater with ulceration and bleeding.

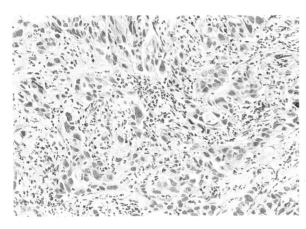

C. Biopsy demonstrating a poorly differentiated adenocarcinoma. H.E., x 200

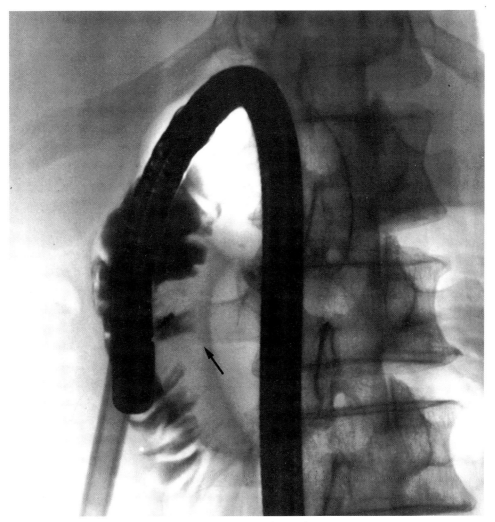

D. Endoscopic retrograde cholangiopancreatogram (ERCP) showing an obstruction of the main
pancreatic duct (MPD) at the head (arrow) due to a space-occupying lesion in the pancreatic
head.

Case 16   Cancer of the papilla of Vater due to invasion from cancer of the pancreatic head

A 48-year-old male with a history of diabetes mellitus. *Chief complaints:* right upper quadrant pain and fever (38–39°C). *Treatment:* cholecystoduodenostomy and gastrojejunostomy.

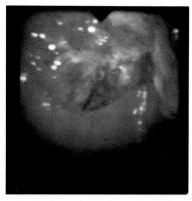 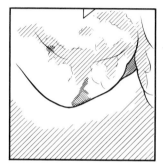

A. Duodenoscopy revealing a large ulcer with a dirty yellowish covering and bleeding surrounded by a wall at the area of the papilla of Vater.

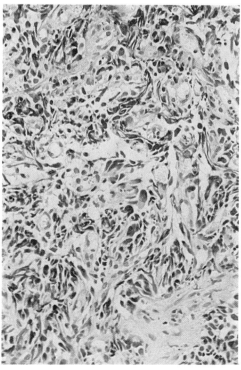

B. Biopsy demonstrating a poorly differentiated adenocarcinoma. H.E., x 200

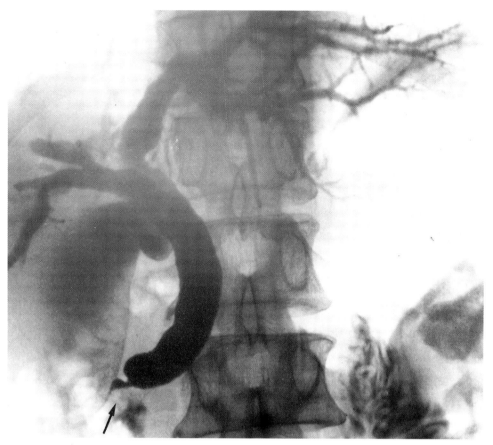

C. ERC with no visualized pancreatic duct and a defect (arrow) at the lower margin of the ampulla of Vater.

5

Endoscopic Retrograde Cholangiopancreatography

TATSUZO KASUGAI, M.D.

Endoscopic retrograde cholangiopancreatography (ERCP) is performed with a fiberscope by injecting contrast material through a cannula inserted into the ampulla through the orifice of the papilla of Vater under direct vision.

ERCP is one of the most reliable procedures for detecting disorders of the pancreaticobiliary system.

Indications and Contraindications

This procedure is indicated for the diagnosis of diseases of the pancreas, biliary system and liver, as shown in Table 5-1.

The contraindications for ERCP include those previously mentioned as contraindications for upper gastrointestinal (GI) endoscopy. Patients with severe illness may not tolerate endoscopy. Poor risk patients, those with infectious diseases, acute cholangitis and patients in whom an endoscope could not be inserted should be excluded. Therefore, an evaluation of the general condition for tolerating an endoscopy, and an upper GI series to check for a stenosis or deformity in the upper GI tract that might prevent instrumentation should be done before proceeding with an ERCP.

The procedure must be carefully performed in patients with iodine allergy and in

Table 5-1 Indications for ERCP *.

Jaundice, obscure etiology
Probable stones in biliary system not demonstrable by ordinary X-ray methods
Malignancy of hepatobiliary system and of the pancreas
Pancreatitis, chronic, doubtful
Pancreatic tumors, including cysts
Extrinsic compression of stomach and/or duodenum on X-ray or endoscopy
Diabetes mellitus with abdominal complaints and weight loss to rule out pancreatitis or pancreatic carcinoma
Peripapillary duodenal diverticulum with symptoms
Gastric cancer with probable pancreatic invasion
Metastatic adenocarcinoma, primary site undetermined, possibly biliary or pancreatic
Patients with upper abdominal complaints and no demonstrable lesions in stomach, duodenum, or liver

* From Kasugai, T., Kuno, N., and Kizu, M.: Manometric endoscopic retrograde pancreatocholangiography. Technique, significance, and evaluation. Amer. J. Digest. Dis. 19: 485-502, 1974.

those who are allergic to contrast material. However, the procedure can be safely done if special care is given in those patients who have been allergic to contrast material given for intravenous cholangiography.

Those with acute pancreatitis, however, are excluded because of the possibility that an increase in the pancreatic duct pressure might aggravate the condition. In chronic relapsing pancreatitis the procedure can be done by avoiding the relapsing stage. Patients with HBsAg are excluded because of possible dissemination of the virus. If the procedure is requested, it should be done as the last case of an ERCP session on the same day taking special precautions to prevent infection. The fiberscope and other equipment should be strictly sterilized with 2 percent glutaraldehyde solution or ethylene oxide gas after the procedure.

Other imagings such as ultrasonography, CT scanning and radioisotope scintigraphy should be selectively performed as a screening procedure before ERCP or as a precise examination depending upon the disease or the case.

Instruments

Side-viewing fiberscopes such as JF type B4 and Fujinon QB are used for cannulation into the ampulla of Vater.

Occasionally forward-viewing fiberscopes such as GIF type Q or P3 are preferable for cannulation in cases of post-operative stomach with Billroth II anastomosis.

Premedication and post endoscopy care of patients are described in Chapter 1.

Technique

A close-up en face view of the papilla of Vater should be obtained and then a cannula inserted into the orifice. The cannula must be inserted vertically — to right from left in the visual field — into the ampulla of Vater to visualize the pancreatic duct and should be inserted into the ampulla superficially upward, almost parallel with the longitudinal fold — to left from right in the visual field — to opacify the biliary system. To fill both duct systems, the cannula should be inserted only 5–6 mm into the duct. As a rule, the cannula is relatively superficially inserted, usually about 10 to 20 mm, and not more than about 30 mm. In cases with two separate orifices, selective cannulation of each orifice should be carried out.

If the tip presses against the duct wall, satisfactory visualization of the duct system cannot be obtained in spite of a high pressure. In such instances, reinsertion should be tried. A schematic drawing of various shapes of the papilla of Vater and its orifices is shown in Figure 5-1.

To prevent infectious complications after ERCP, sterilization is essential. The duodenoscope and its biopsy channel should be washed repeatedly with soap solution followed by 2 percent glutaraldehyde solution and water, and the manometer and cannula are sterilized with ethylene oxide gas. We recommend routine administration of antibiotics or chemotherapeutic agents, both systemically and mixed with the contrast material. In addition, when the pancreas has been heavily opacified by contrast material with excessive acinar filling, it is desirable to use an enzyme inhibitor such as Trasylol or FOY (Gabexate mesilate).

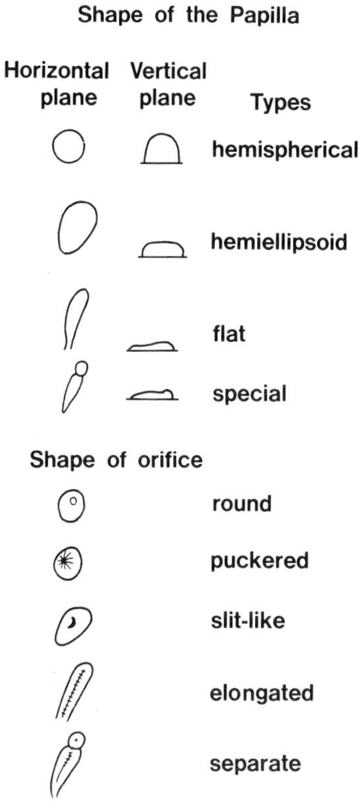

Shape of the Papilla

Fig. 5-1 Various shapes of the papilla of Vater and duct orifices.

Pancreatic Carcinoma

The findings of pancreatic carcinoma consist of a stricture of varying extent and degree, obstruction or abruption, and displacement of the main pancreatic duct (MPD), and rigidity, dilatation, stenosis, obstruction and irregular distribution of branches of the pancreatic duct and fine pancreatic ducts (FPD). In addition, pancreatic field defects are seen. These are due to compression, displacement, and defects of branches, FPD, and acini. The pancreatic field is normally formed by the shadows of branches, FPD, and occasionally acini.

Coarse acinar opacification and pooling of contrast material are also found occasionally.

In cases with opacified biliary systems only, displacement, irregular stricture, defects, and complete or incomplete obstruction of the lower portions of the common bile duct with dilated proximal bile ducts are observed.

Pancreatic carcinoma in ERCP is classified into four types as shown in Figure 5-2.

Chronic Pancreatitis

The revised criteria listed for ERCP diagnosis of chronic pancreatitis (Table 5-2) have been proposed on the basis of our early ERCP studies combined with postmortem pancreatograms (PMP) and finally confirmed by microscopic examination of the pancreas.

Table 5-2 Criteria for ERCP diagnosis of chronic pancreatitis *.

	Pancreatitis stage		
	Minimal (MIP)	Moderate (MOP)	Advanced (ADP)
Pancreas			
Main pancreatic duct (MPD)			
Rigidity	$-\sim\pm$	$+\sim++$	$+\sim++$
Tortuosity	$-\sim\pm$	$+\sim++$	$++\sim+++$
Dilatation and stenosis	$-$	$+$	$++\sim+++$
Obstruction	$-$	$-$	$+$
Cyst formation	$-$	$-$	$+$
Calculi	$-$	$-$	$+$
Branches and fine pancreatic ducts (FPD)			
Rigidity	$+$	$+\sim++$	$+\sim++$
Irregular distribution	$+$	$+\sim++$	$+\sim+++$
Dilatation	$+$	$+\sim++$	$+\sim+++$
Stenosis and obstruction	$+$	$+\sim++$	$+\sim+++$
Cystic dilatation	$+$	$+$	$+\sim+++$
Calculi	$-$	$-$	$+$
Acini			
Coarse opacification	$-$	$-$	$+$
Size of pancreas			
Diminished	$-$	$-$	$+$
Biliary system			
Pancreatic portion			
Rigidity	$-$	$+$	$+\sim+++$
Dilatation	$-$	$+$	$+\sim++$
Stenosis	$-$	$+$	$-\sim+++$
Defect and obstruction	$-$	$-$	$+$

* From Kasugai, T., Kuno, N., and Kizu, M.: Manometric endoscopic retrograde pancreatocholangiography. Technique, significance, and evaluation. Amer. J. Digest. Dis.
19: 485-502, 1974.

Chronic pancreatitis cases are graded based on these criteria as minimal (MIP),
moderate (MOP), and advanced chronic pancreatitis (ADP).

Correlations between pancreatograms obtained on the autopsied pancreas and the
microscopic findings are presented in Figure 5-3.

Of 32 cases interpreted as normal PMP, 23 (71.9%) showed histologically normal
findings. Of 19 cases diagnosed as MIP in PMP, 18 (94.7%) were interpreted histologically as chronic pancreatitis, and 15 (78.9%) were diagnosed as MIP. All the 21 cases
interpreted as MOP in PMP showed chronic inflammation histologically, and 18
(85.7%) of them had MOP. The six cases of ADP in PMP had advanced chronic inflammation microscopically. 71.9 percent of cases interpreted as normal and 97.8 percent
of cases diagnosed as chronic pancreatitis in PMP showed histologically normal or
chronic pancreatitis respectively.

A positive correlation of the severity of inflammation in both examinations was
noted in 62 of 78 cases (79.5%).

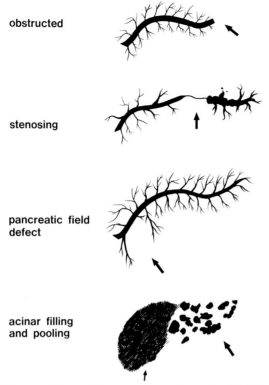

Fig. 5-2 Types of pancreatic carcinoma in ERCP.

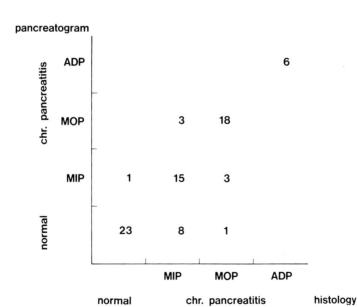

Fig. 5-3 Correlation between postmortem pancreatograms (PMP) and histology in 78 cases.

ERCP seems to be a reliable morphologic diagnostic method, because there was an 80 percent positive correlation in quantitative interpretation.

Hereafter, correlative studies between pancreatograms and microscopic interpretation will require a large number of cases for statistical analysis.

ERCP and PTC

ERCP and percutaneous transhepatic cholangiography (PTC) are complementary techniques for examination of the biliary tract. Using either or both techniques most cases of extrahepatic biliary obstruction can now be diagnosed precisely prior to surgery.

Endoscopic Sphincterotomy (EST)

Endoscopic sphincterotomy (EST) has been performed safely with a diathermy knife introduced via a duodenoscope to remove common duct stones (see Chapter 6).

Complications associated with ERCP and their Prevention

Complications in 3 percent, and death in 0.2 percent among 10,435 examinations for ERCP were reported by Bilbao et al.

The complications included pancreatitis, cholangitis, pancreatic sepsis, instrumental injury to the gastrointestinal tract, and drug reactions. Pancreatitis was associated with injection into the pancreatic duct, sepsis with injection into an obstructed duct or pseudocyst, and injury with abnormal gastroduodenal anatomy.

The complications associated with ERCP in Japan have been evaluated (Table 5-3).

Specific data on complications were reported for 60,960 ERCP's and formed the basis of the complications that follow. "Successes" were reported in 55,140 cases (90.5%); complications occurred in 479 (0.78%); death in 75 (0.12%); emergency admission in 345 (0.57%); emergency laparotomy in 59 (0.097%).

Table 5-3 Complications of ERCP in Japan (March 26, 1978). Total examinations 60,960 (successful cannulations 55,140)

Complication	No. of cases	Incidence (%)	Deaths	Fatality rate (%)
Cholangitis	213	0.39	45	0.08
Pancreatitis	134	0.24	7	0.01
Instrumental injury	39	0.06	6	0.01
Pancreatic sepsis, pseudocyst, abscess	30	0.05	5	0.009
Drug reaction	19	0.03	1	0.002
Peritonitis of unknown causes	9	0.015	3	0.005
Cardio-pulmonary	7	0.01	3	0.005
Aspiration pneumonia	1	0.002		
Acute hepatitis	1	0.002	1	0.002
Miscellaneous	26	0.04	4	0.007
Total	479	0.78	75	0.12

Morbidity : 479/60960 (0.78 %)　Mortality : 75/60960 (0.12%)

Complications included 213 cases (0.39%) of cholangitis, 134 (0.24%) of pancreatitis, 39 (0.06%) of instrumental injury to the gastrointestinal tract, 30 (0.05%) of pancreatic sepsis, pseudocyst and abscess, 19 of drug reactions, 9 of peritonitis of unknown causes and 7 of cardio-pulmonary diseases.

There were 75 deaths (0.12%), 45 (0.08%) had cholangitis, 7 (0.01%) had pancreatitis, 6 (0.01%) had instrumental injury and 5 (0.009%) had pancreatic sepsis, pseudocyst or abscess.

For experienced workers the incidence of complications was 0.4 percent whereas in the inexperienced it was three times greater (1.3%). In general, inexperienced workers had a relatively higher incidence of complications than experienced workers.

Six hundred and eight endoscopic sphincterotomies have been performed at 34 centers in Japan and 43 (7.1%) complications were encountered. The complications included 17 cases of hemorrhage, 9 of pancreatitis, 8 of cholangitis, 3 of perforation and 4 of restenosis and others. Two (0.3%) fatal complications were associated with endoscopic sphincterotomy, one with cholangitis and one with liver abscess.

Endoscopic collection of pancreatic juice has been studied in 886 cases at 16 centers in Japan, with only one case of pancreatitis as a complication.

One hundred and eighty-two cholangiopancreatoscopies have been performed by peroral endoscopy at 6 centers and no complications have been reported.

For prevention of ERCP complications we must practice the following procedures as shown in Table 5-4; special training programs in ERCP to lower the incidence of ERCP complications in experienced workers, strict indications, cautious premedication, attempt to avoid infection and sepsis, i.e., 1) disinfection of instruments used in ERCP, 2) make a clean examination and use aseptic procedures as much as possible, 3) prophylactic antibiotic use, 4) antibiotics mixed with contrast medium, and 5) administration of antibiotics, before, during and after the examination, if necessary. The above points are most important for preventing serious complications. Moreover, we recommend the use of a manometer to measure and control the injection pressure of the contrast medium, decompression by PTC-drainage or early surgery, if necessary, and administration of antienzyme, if necessary when heavy parenchymal opacification of the pancreas is obtained.

Table 5-4 Prevention of ERCP complications.

1. Special training programs in ERCP
2. Strict indication
3. Cautious premedication
4. Disinfection of instruments
5. Attempt to avoid sepsis (clean examination)
6. Prophylactic antibiotic use
7. Antibiotics mixed with contrast medium
8. Administration of antibiotics, before, during, and after the examination, if necessary
9. Measure and control of injection pressure of contrast medium
10. Decompression by PTC-drainage or early surgery, if necessary
11. Administration of antienzyme, if necessary

REFERENCES

1) Bilbao, M.K., Dotter, C.T., Lee, T.G., and Katon, R.M.: Complication of endoscopic retrograde cholangiopancreatography. Gastroenterology 70: 314-320, 1976.
2) Kasugai, T., Kuno, N., and Kizu, M.: Manometric endoscopic retrograde pancreatocholangiography. Technique, significance, and evaluation. Amer. J. Digest. Dis. 19: 485-502, 1974.
3) Kasugai, T.: Recent advances in the endoscopic retrograde cholangiopancreatography. Digestion 13: 76-99, 1975.
4) Kasugai, T.: ERCP — complications and its prevention. Rinsho geka 33: 1533-1541, 1978 (in Japanese)
5) Kasugai, T.: Indications and contraindications for endoscopic retrograde cholangiopancreatography. In: Takemoto, T. and Kasugai, T. (eds.) Endoscopic retrograde cholangiopancreatography, p. 32, Igaku-Shoin, Tokyo, 1979.
6) Kasugai, T.: Pancreatits. In Takemoto, T. and Kasugai, T. (eds.) Endoscopic retrograde cholangiopancreatography, pp. 176-202, Igaku-Shoin, Tokyo, 1979.

Case 1 Normal endoscopic retrograde cholangiopancreatograms (ERCP)

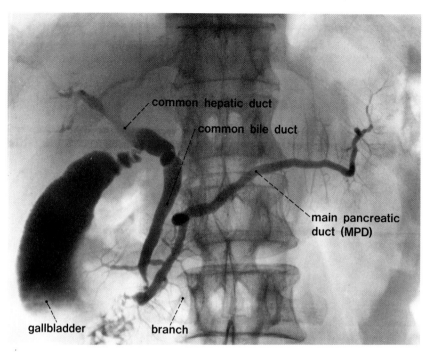

A. Normal ERCP, branch opacification.

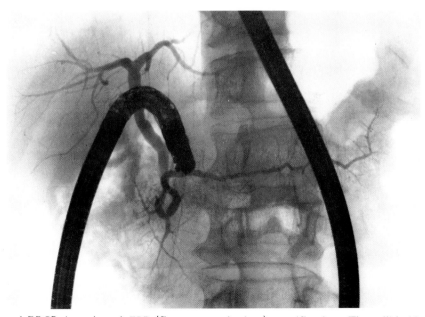

B. Normal ERCP, branch and FPD (fine pancreatic duct) opacification. The gallbladder is not visualized due to cholecystectomy.

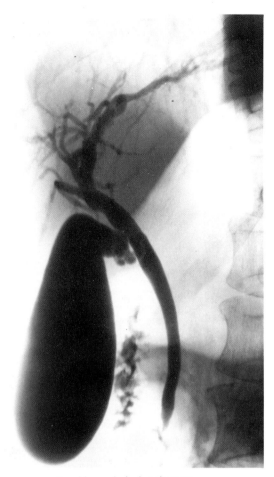

C.   Normal cholangiogram.

Case 2   Cancer of the tail of the pancreas : obstructed type

A 75-year-old male. *Chief complaints:* epigastric pain and back pain. Pancreatic juice was collected during cannulation of the ampulla of Vater and the cytology demonstrated adenocarcinoma cells.

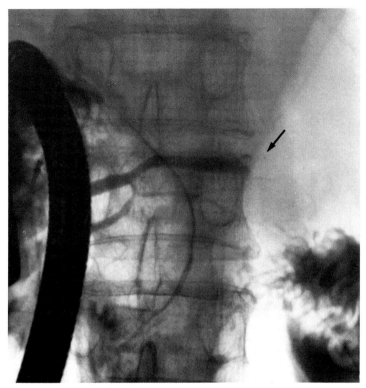

Endoscopic retrograde pancreatogram (ERP) revealing an obscure, dull abruption of the main pancreatic duct (MPD) between the body and tail of the pancreas (arrow).

Case 3   Cancer of the pancreatic body : stenosing type

A 54-year-old male. *Chief complaint:* epigastric pain.

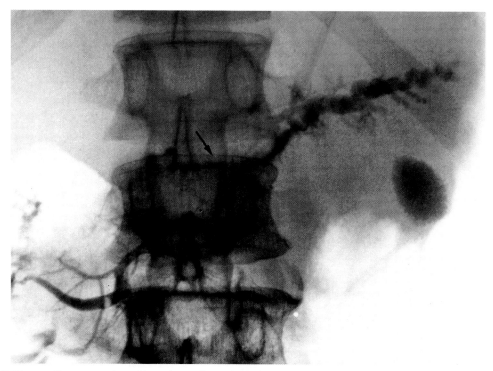

ERP revealing marked stricture (arrow) of the MPD in the body with irregularly dilated MPD and branches in the tail of the pancreas.

Case 4 Cancer of the pancreatic head mainly in the uncus area : pancreatic field defect type

A 33-year-old male. *Chief complaints:* epigastric pain and weight loss.

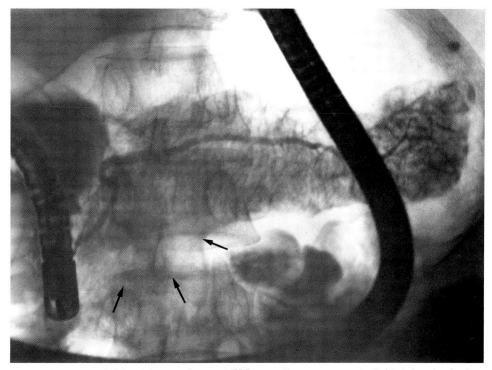

ERP visualizing the MPD with branches and FPD revealing a pancreatic field defect in the lower part of the pancreatic head, mainly in the uncus area (arrow), while the MPD remains normal.

Case 5 Cancer of the entire pancreas : acinar filling and pooling type

A 63-year-old female. *Chief complaint:* epigastric mass.

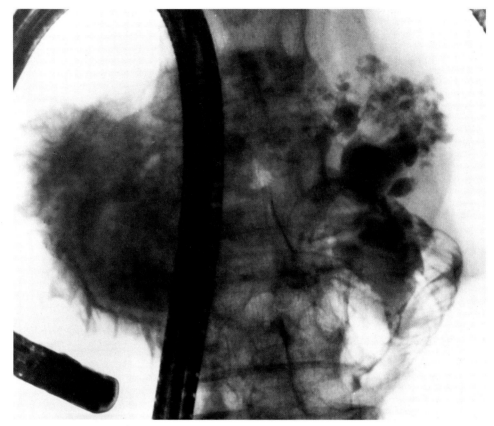

ERP revealing a coarse acinar filling in the head and body of the pancreas, and many pools of contrast material of varying size in the tail, with obstructed MPD in the head.

Case 6 Chronic pancreatitis : minimal pancreatitis (MIP)

A 63-year-old male. *Chief complaints:* abdominal fullness and back pain. He had a history of cholelithiasis. *Treatment:* cholecystectomy and medical treatment.

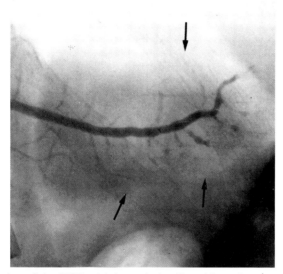

ERP revealing tortuosity of the MPD with irregularly dilated branches (arrows) in the tail of the pancreas.

Case 7   Chronic pancreatitis : moderate pancreatitis (MOP)

A 62-year-old male. *Chief complaints:* dull epigastric pain and back pain.

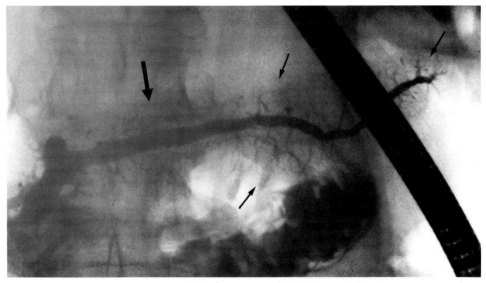

ERP revealing an irregularly dilated MPD (large arrow) with irregularly dilated branches (small arrows).

Case 8 Chronic pancreatitis : moderate pancreatitis (MOP)

A 68-year-old male. *Chief complaints:* fatigue and jaundice. His primary disease was cancer of the common hepatic duct.

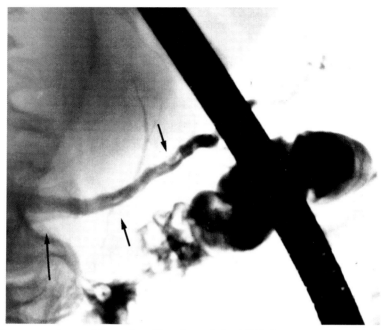

ERP revealing tortuosity and irregular dilatation of the MPD (long arrow) and irregular cable-like radiolucencies (short arrows) at the tail of the MPD which suggest the existence of protein plugs.

Case 9   Chronic pancreatitis : advanced pancreatitis (ADP)

A 67-year-old female. *Chief complaint:* fatigue.

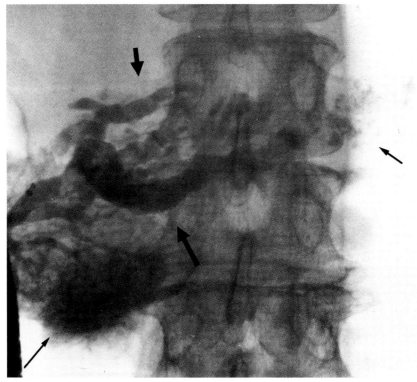

ERP revealing markedly irregular dilatation of the MPD (long, large arrow) which is abrupted at the tail due to calculi (short, small arrow) with markedly irregular dilated branches (short, large arrow). A long, small arrow indicates coarse acinar filling.

Case 10   Chronic pancreatitis : advanced pancreatitis (ADP)

A 68-year-old female. *Chief complaint:* epigastric pain.

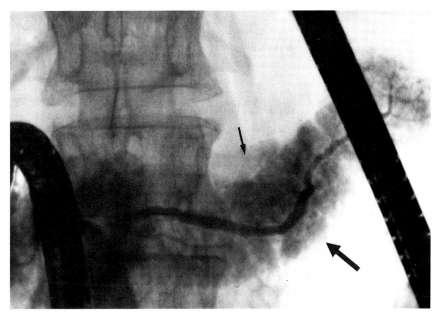

A.   ERP revealing marked tortuosity and segmental dilatation (large arrow) of the MPD with dilated branches and coarse acinar filling (small arrow).

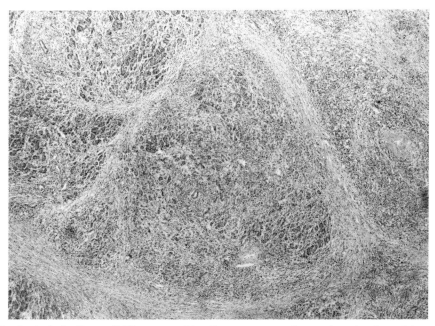

B.   Histological findings. Diffuse atrophic disappearance of exocrine glands and intra- and interlobular marked fibrosis with severe infiltration of plasma cells and lymphocytes are observed. ADP and so-called pancreatic sclerosis. H.E., x 10

Case 11 **True pancreatic cyst**

A 33-year-old female. *Chief complaint:* a palpable tumor in the left upper quadrant. *Treatment:* resection of the tail of the pancreas.

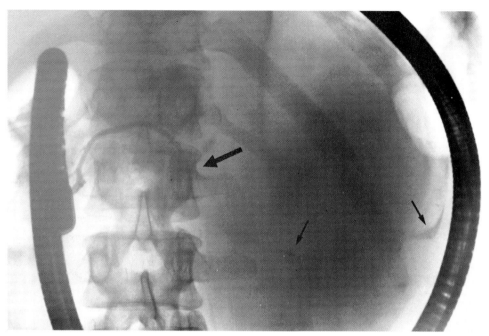

A. There is downward displacement, compression, and a tapering stricture of the MPD at the beginning of the body (large arrow), and marked downward displacement and compression of remaining MPD showing an irregular narrowing and dilatation in the body and tail of the pancreas (small arrows). These findings suggest the existence of a huge mass in the body and tail of the pancreas. (From Kasugai, T., Kuno, N., and Kizu, M.: Manometric endoscopic retrograde pancreatocholangiography. Technique, significance, and evaluation. Amer. J. Digest. Dis. 19: 485-502, 1974.)

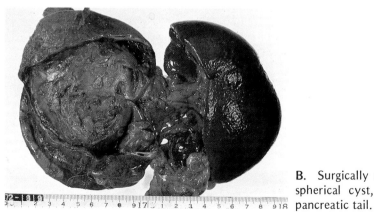

B. Surgically resected specimen showing a spherical cyst, 12 cm in diameter, in the pancreatic tail.

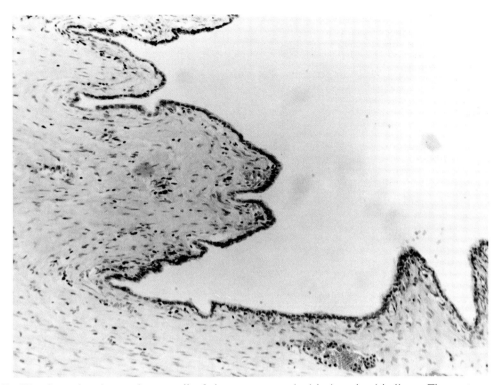

C. Histology showing an inner wall of the cyst covered with ductal epithelium. The cyst may be formed from a cystic dilatation of the pancreatic duct. True pancreatic cyst. H.E., x 20

Case 12   Pseudopancreatic cyst

A 73-year-old female. *Chief complaints:* right upper quadrant pain and jaundice. Her primary disease was cancer of the common bile duct.

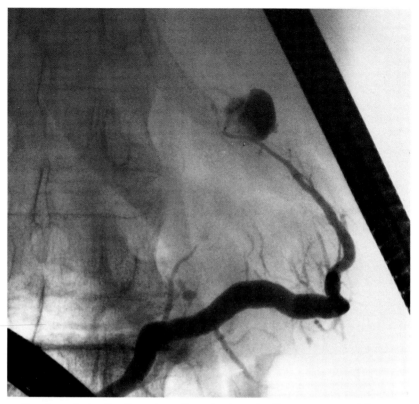

ERCP revealing irregularly distributed medium-sized pools of contrast material, connected with the irregularly dilated MPD in the pancreatic tail.

Case 13 Trauma of the pancreas

A 45-year-old male. *Chief complaint:* epigastric pain immediately after a blow to the abdomen in a traffic accident. *Treatment:* resection of the pancreatic body and tail.

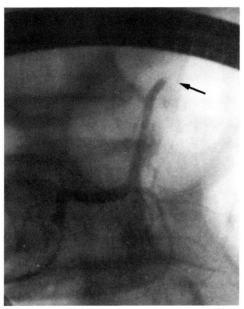

ERP revealing an abruption of the MPD (arrow) between the head and body of the pancreas. (Courtesy of Dr. D. Hirooka)

Case 14   Cholelithiasis

A 54-year-old female. *Chief complaint:* epigastric pain. *Treatment:* cholecystectomy. Stone, 4.0 x 2.5 x 2.5 cm.

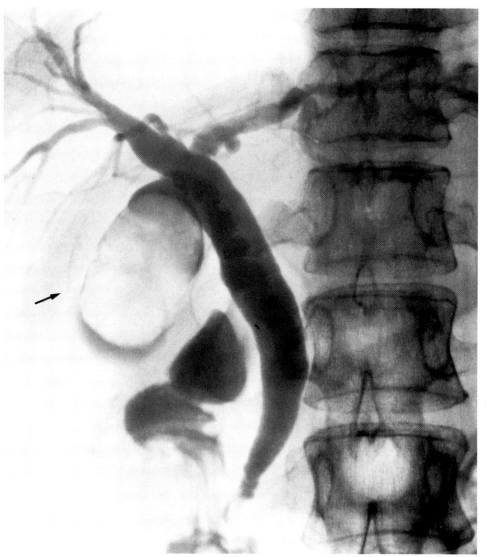

Endoscopic retrograde cholangiogram (ERC) revealing a huge radiolucency, 4.0 x 2.8 cm in size, in the gallbladder.

Case 15 Choledochocholelithiasis

A 68-year-old female. *Chief complaints:* right upper quadrant pain and right back pain.

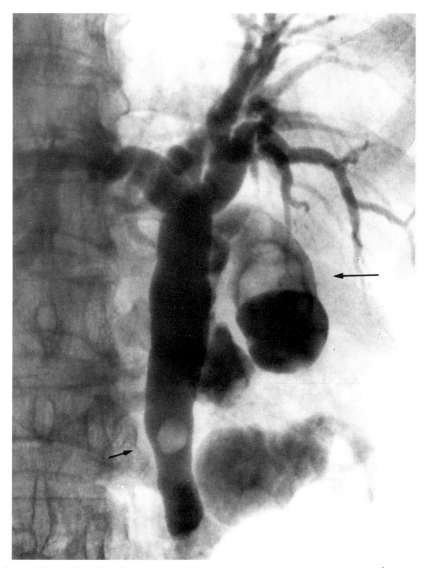

ERC taken with patient in the prone position revealing many radiolucencies (long arrow) of various size in the gallbladder and a round radiolucency (short arrow) in the dilated common bile duct.

Case 16   Choledocholithiasis with stones in the liver

A 66-year-old male. *Chief complaint:* colicky pain attack in the epigastric region. *Treatment:* cholecystectomy, choledocholithotomy and choledochoduodenostomy.

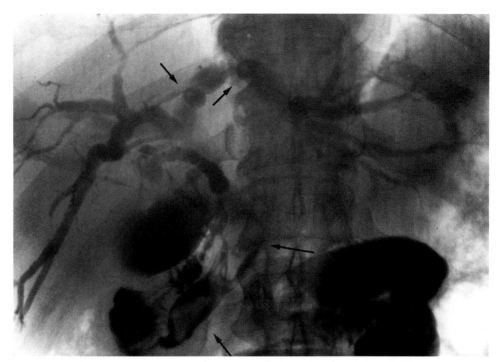

ERC showing two large radiolucencies (long arrows) in the dilated common bile duct and many small radiolucencies (short arrows) in the dilated hepatic ducts and intrahepatic bile ducts.

Case 17 Choledochocholelithiasis with stones in the liver

A 53-year-old male. *Chief complaint:* colicky pain in the epigastrium. *Treatment:* cholecystectomy, cholangiolithotomy and choledochoduodenostomy.

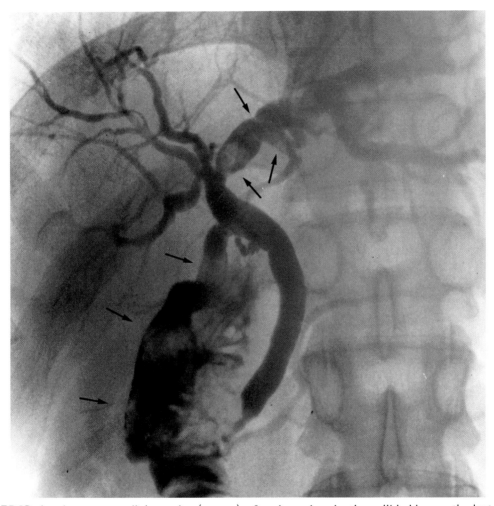

ERCP showing many radiolucencies (arrows) of various sizes in the gallbladder, cystic duct, dilated hepatic duct and intrahepatic bile ducts.

Case 18   Cancer of the common bile duct

A 66-year-old male. *Chief complaint:* jaundice. *Treatment:* choledochectomy, chole-cystectomy and choledochojejunostomy.

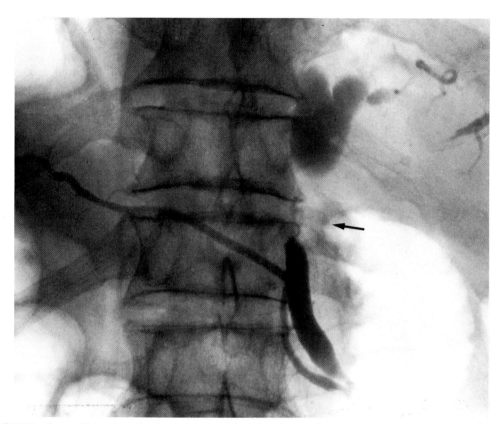

ERCP taken with patient in the prone position showing an incomplete obstruction (arrow) at the confluence of three ducts (the common bile duct, common hepatic duct and cystic duct) with dilated proximal common hepatic duct and hepatic ducts.

Case 19 Cancer of the common bile duct with metastases in lymph nodes of the porta hepatis

A 70-year-old male. *Chief complaint:* jaundice.

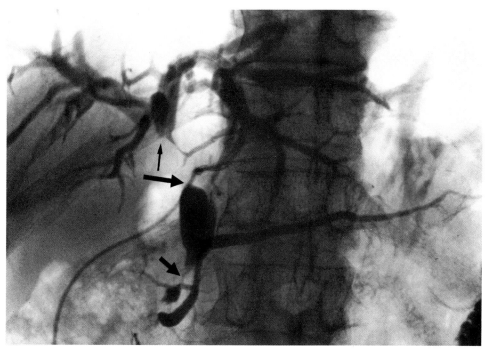

ERCP revealing an irregular stricture in the common bile duct (short, large arrow) and a complete obstruction of the extrahepatic bile duct at the level of the confluence of the three ducts (long, large arrow), and PTC showing a tapering obstruction of the common hepatic duct at the level of the porta hepatis (short, small arrow). This cholangiogram was taken by means of both procedures of ERCP and PTC performed simultaneously.

Case 20   Cancer of the common hepatic duct

A 75-year-old male. *Chief complaints:* jaundice and nausea. *Treatment:* cholangioectomy and cholangioduodenostomy.

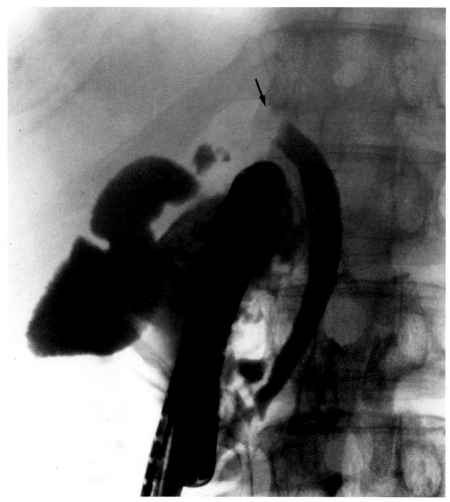

ERC revealing an abruption of the common hepatic duct with irregular ending (arrow), with the incompletely obstructed cystic duct. (From Kasugai, T., Kuno, N., and Kizu, M.: Endoscopic pancreatocholangiography with special reference to manometric method. Med. J. Aust. 2: 717-725, 1973.)

Case 21 Cancer of the gallbladder with choledocholithiasis

A 79-year-old male. *Chief complaints:* right upper quadrant pain and nausea.

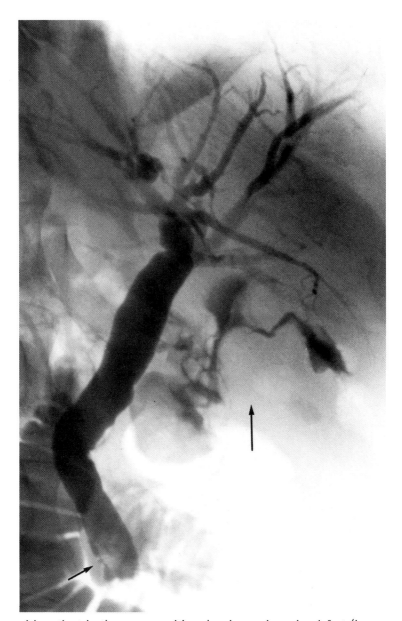

ERC taken with patient in the prone position showing an irregular defect (long arrow) in the gallbladder and an irregular radiolucency (short arrow) at the distal portion of the dilated common bile duct.

Case 22   Liver abscess with choledocholithiasis

A 51-year-old female. *Chief complaints:* right upper quadrant pain and occasional fever. *Treatment:* choledocholithotomy and hepatotomy.

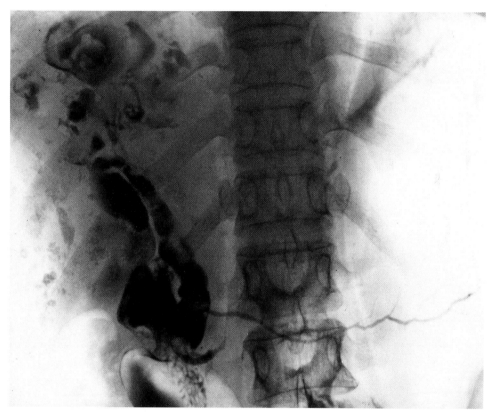

ERCP revealing several irregularly oval radiolucencies in the dilated common bile duct and common hepatic duct and multiple irregularly shaped pooling of contrast material like petals of various sizes connecting with dilated intrahepatic bile ducts in the liver. (From Kasugai, T., Kuno, N., and Kizu, M.: Endoscopic pancreatocholangiography with special reference to manometric method. Med. J. Aust. 2: 717-725, 1973.)

Case 23   Primary sclerosing cholangitis

A 38-year-old male. *Chief complaint:* jaundice with disturbance of liver function. He
has suffered from ulcerative colitis for ten years.

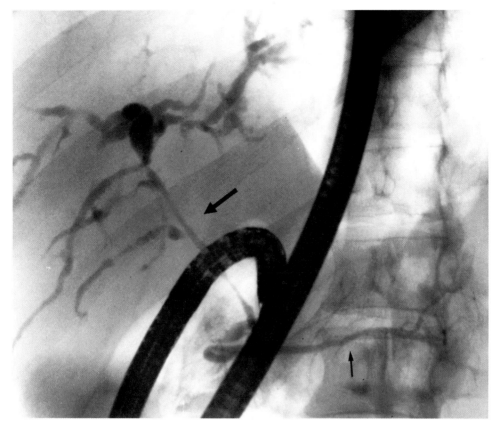

ERCP revealing a markedly irregular narrowing of the common bile duct and the lower and
mid-portions of the common hepatic duct (large arrow), and partial dilatation of the common
hepatic duct at the level of the porta hepatis and moderate dilatation or partial stenosis of the
hepatic ducts and intrahepatic bile ducts with rigidity of the walls. A small arrow indicates
the MPD. (Courtesy of Dr. R.J. Fitch)

Case 24 Malformation of the biliary system : anomalous arrangement of the biliary and pancreatic ducts

A 24-year-old female. *Chief complaint:* colicky pain attack in the epigastrium. *Treatment:* choledochoduodenostomy.

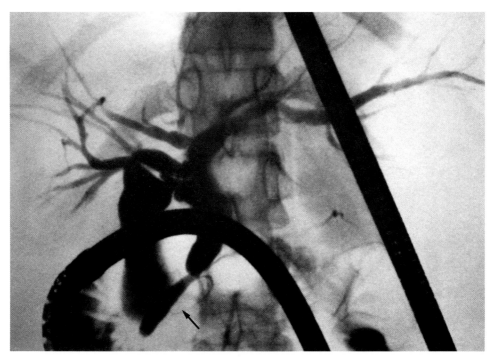

ERCP revealing a slightly dilated common bile duct, 12 mm in diameter, coming down into the MPD at the portion between the head and body of the pancreas and a markedly dilated portion of the MPD in the head, 8 mm in diameter, is regarded to be a long common channel, 37 mm in length.

6

Endoscopic Sphincterotomy (EST) of the Papilla of Vater

MASATSUGU NAKAJIMA, M.D. and KEIICHI KAWAI, M.D.

Great advances in fiberoptic duodenoscopy, especially the ability to pass instruments through an endoscope into the papilla of Vater, have led to the widespread use of endoscopic retrograde cholangiopancreatography (ERCP) in the diagnosis and management of biliary and pancreatic diseases. The logical extension of this technical facility has also opened a new possibility for endoscopic biliary tract surgery. This is endoscopic sphincterotomy (EST) of the papilla of Vater, which combines and modifies the techniques of endoscopic retrograde cannulation and diathermic electrosurgery. Within only several years of its development, this new surgical endoscopy has become an acceptable alternative to transabdominal surgery for treatment of biliary tract diseases, especially for stones. Recently, the techniques, instruments and indications for EST have rapidly evolved.

Instrumentation

EST is made possible by the combined use of an insulated side-viewing duodenoscope for retrograde instrumentation of the bile duct and an electrode catheter (sphincterotome) for section of the sphincter of Oddi. Figure 6-1 shows our latest improved electrode catheter for sphincterotomy. It is 1,850 mm long with an external diameter of 1.7 mm, and it can pass through an instrument channel of a duodenoscope. This sphincterotome consists of a diathermic wire, housed within a single teflon sheath, with the distal 20 mm of wire exposed and fixed at the tip. The free end of the wire is attached to the adjusting handle which is connected to an electrosurgical unit. This is designed so that the sphincter of Oddi can be sectioned by selectively pushing or pulling the diathermic wire exposed at the tip. It is also possible to inject contrast medium through the catheter for opacifying the bile and pancreatic ducts.

Techniques

The procedure is done in the X-ray room with access to fluoroscopy. Under topical pharyngeal anesthesia and intravenous premedication for sedation and duodenal atony, the tip of the electrode catheter (sphincterotome) is selectively cannulated through a duodenoscope into the distal common bile duct, not into the pancreatic duct, in a manner similar to ERCP. EST is performed by selectively pushing or pulling the diathermic wire exposed at the tip of the sphincterotome and by intermittently and repeatedly discharging a high frequency current for cutting (Fig. 6-2). The safe electrosurgical section of the sphincter should be limited to the proximal end of the roof of the papilla visualized through an endoscope. Complete or total sphincterotomy

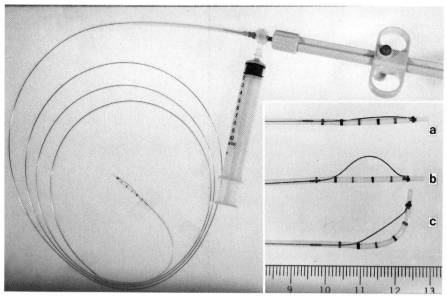

Fig. 6-1 Wire-tipped sphincterotome now in use for EST. This is designed so that the diather-mic cutting wire exposed at the tip(a) can be selectively pushed(b) or pulled(c) to section the sphincter by manipulating the adjusting handle.

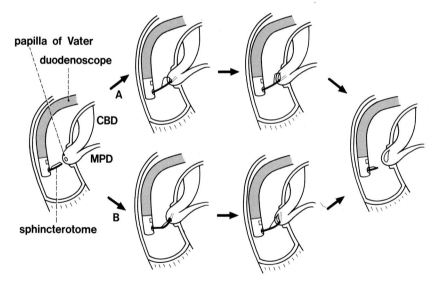

Fig. 6-2 Techniques of EST. A: wire-pushing technique with a pulsion-type sphincterotome, B: wire-pulling technique with a traction-type sphincterotome. CBD, common bile duct; MPD, main pancreatic duct. (From Nakajima, M. et al.: Endoscopic sphincterotomy (EST) of the papilla of Vater: Its technique, significance and evaluation. In: Takemoto, T. and Kasugai, T. (eds.) Endoscopic Retrograde Cholangiopancreatography, pp. 73-93, Igaku-Shoin, Tokyo, 1979.)

including the section of the superior sphincter extending above the intramural portion of the distal common bile duct often produces retroperitoneal leakage, which may develop into a serious complication. After an adequate EST, the superior sphincter of the distal common bile duct remains, but may be functionally effaced. The temporary wound produced by the sphincterotomy heals within a week, forming a terminal biliary fistula. ERCP is repeated one or two weeks after the procedure to evaluate the effects of EST.

Removal of Stones

Following successful EST, biliary tract stones are removed by two processes. The one is spontaneous passage of stones which is facilitated by the use of cholagogues. Most stones, especially those less than 10 mm in size, pass spontaneously within one or two weeks after EST, if the sphincter is adequately sectioned. The other is direct manipulative extraction of stones by using a basket-tipped catheter (Fig. 6-3). A basket-tipped catheter passed through an endoscope is easily introduced into the biliary tract following EST and it is advanced over stones. After opening the basket, the catheter is gradually and gently withdrawn to catch a stone under fluoroscopic control. After successfully catching and ensnaring a stone, the catheter is then pulled out with a little more force to extract it.

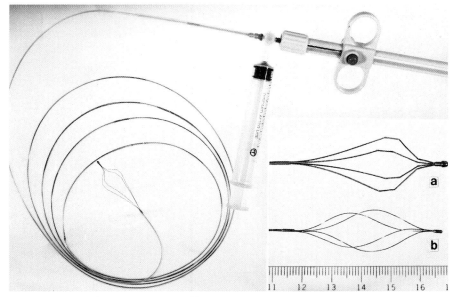

Fig. 6-3 Two types of basket-tipped catheters for extracting stones. a: soft basket, b: hard basket.

Patient Selection and Results

During the last seven years from 1973, EST was accomplished in 263 patients and failed in 7 patients because of technical or anatomical limitations (Table 6-1). Of 245 patients with biliary tract stones in whom EST was performed, the stones were completely removed in 235 patients (95.5%); in 77 patients by spontaneous passage, in 122

Table 6-1 Results of EST attempted in 270 patients.

Indications	No. of patients	Success of EST	Effects of EST	
Cholelithiasis	251	245	235:	Removal of stones*
Choledocholithiasis after cholecystectomy	(153)	(148)	(141)	
Choledocholithiasis in high operative risk patients	(66)	(65)	(63)	
Cholecystocholedocholithiasis scheduled for surgery	(28)	(28)	(28)	
Intrahepatic biliary tract stones	(4)	(4)	(3)	
Benign stenosis of the papilla of Vater	15	14	14:	Obviation of cholestasis
Tumor of the biliary tract	4	4	4:	For PCS** and biopsy
Total	270	263 (95.5%)	253 (93.7%)	

```
*    Spontaneous passage           :  77
     Basket retrieval              : 122
     Combined use of both processes :  36
**   Peroral cholangioscopy
```

patients by basket retrieval and in 36 patients by the combined use of both processes. The size of stones removed following EST ranged from 5 to 45 mm, mostly between 10 and 20 mm. In the other 10 patients, removal of stones was incomplete because of the multiplicity and size of the stones. In patients with choledocholithiasis with or without an intact gallbladder who were judged unfit for laparotomy because of their poor operative risk, no cholecystectomy was attempted following EST and removal of common bile duct stones. On the other hand, in patients with cholecystocholedocholithiasis scheduled for transabdominal surgery, only simple cholecystectomy without choledocholithotomy and T-tube drainage was accomplished after complete removal of biliary tract stones by EST. Basket retrieval of stones following EST was successful under direct vision in 3 of 4 patients with intrahepatic cholelithiasis by the use of a specially designed peroral cholangioscope. In 14 of 15 patients with benign stenosis of the papilla, EST also proved to be effective for obviating their cholestasis and symptoms. In 4 patients with biliary tract tumor, direct inspection of the duct and biopsy of the lesion were successful following EST by using a peroral cholangioscope.

Complications

When undertaking this procedure, the following acute or late complications may be considered; 1) duodenal bleeding or perforation that might be produced by too excessive electrosurgical incision, 2) secondary cholangitis or pancreatitis that could be caused by the manipulation, and 3) restenosis of the sphincter of Oddi that might develop from a fibrous constriction or scarring after the sphincterotomy. In our series, 7 acute complications occurred in 263 sphincterotomies (2.7%); 2 of bleeding, 3 of pancreatitis and 2 of septic cholangitis due to stone impaction. In one case of bleeding, emergency laparotomy was performed with good result. However, in one case of septic cholangitis with unsuccessful removal of stones following EST, the patient died because of associated endotoxin shock (mortality rate 0.4%). The remaining 5 were all well managed by conservative therapy. With follow-up observation restenosis of the sphincter has not been observed. Although duodenobiliary reflux of air or gastrointestinal contents has been produced in 75 percent of the patients (including 65 patients with or without an intact gallbladder), no significant late complications such as ascending cholangitis or pancreatitis have been recognized clinically or subclinically. The results apparently show that EST is a safe and effective procedure with a relatively low complication rate when compared with that of the surgical approaches.

Indications and Contraindications

The indications and contraindications for EST are summarized in Table 6-2. The indications for EST are now divided into therapeutic and diagnostic aids owing to the improvement of the techniques and instruments. The first and main indication for therapeutic EST is biliary tract stones, especially residual or recurrent choledocholithiasis after cholecystectomy. In postcholecystectomy patients with residual or recurrent stones and without T-tube drainage or after failure of T-tube stone removal, EST is certainly the procedure of choice prior to a second operation and can eliminate its hazards. In elderly or frail patients with choledocholithiasis and with or without cholecystolithiasis who are judged unfit for laparotomy, the technique will save the patients from the risk of surgery as a temporary maneuver to relieve debilitating cholestasis or sepsis due to biliary tract obstruction. When EST and removal of common bile duct stones were previously successful in patients with cholecystocholedocholithiasis scheduled for laparotomy, only simple cholecystectomy without choledocholithotomy is required at operation, thereby diminishing operating time and difficulty as well as the patients' discomfort. In patients with certain kinds of intrahepatic chole-

Table 6-2 Indications and contraindications for EST.

Indications
Therapeutic: 1. Biliary tract stones
a. Residual or recurrent choledocholithiasis after cholecystectomy
b. Choledocholithiasis with or without an intact gallbladder in poor operative risk patients
c. Cholecystocholedocholithiasis scheduled for transabdominal surgery
d. Intrahepatic biliary tract stones
2. Stenosis of the papilla of Vater
a. Benign stenosis
b. Malignant stenosis
Diagnostic: Any biliary tract disease requiring peroral cholangioscopy and biopsy for precise or differential diagnosis
Contraindications
Pathogenic: 1. Hemorrhagic diathesis
2. Acute pancreatitis
Technical: 1. Long stenosis of the distal common bile duct

lithiasis, direct manipulative extraction of stones is facilitated under direct visual control by the use of a specially designed peroral cholangioscope.

The second therapeutic indication is stenosis of the papilla which does not extend above the intramural portion of the distal common bile duct. EST is effective for obviating its cholestasis and symptoms. The procedure has also been used in patients with a tumor of the papilla of Vater causing distal biliary obstruction, and is a palliative therapy for achieving biliary drainage.

The diagnostic indications for EST are any ductal abnormalities suggesting tumor or inflammation which require further precise diagnosis such as direct endoscopy and biopsy of the ducts. The newly developed technique of peroral cholangioscopy under sliding tube guidance is easily performed following EST and it can provide good visualization of the ductal lumen. It is also possible to take biopsies from the lesions under direct vision. The increasing use of this technique may lead to early detection of tumors of the ducts that may be overlooked or differentiated only with difficulty by conventional methods.

The contraindications for EST are almost the same as those for upper gastrointestinal endoscopy including ERCP. The specific contraindications are listed in Table 6-2. The top two are pathogenetic contraindications and the bottom one is the technical or anatomical one. They must be strictly determined so as not to risk complications as described above.

Conclusion

Endoscopic sphincterotomy (EST), a new concept in therapeutic endoscopy, is now shown to be a practical and relatively safe procedure with a low complication rate when compared with the transabdominal surgical approach. Not only can it be applied in patients unfit for operation, but will lessen the patients' physical discomfort and considerable economic loss associated with removal of stones by established surgical means. The technique has also led to peroral cholangioscopy and transendoscopic instrumentation of the bile duct. The widespread availability of EST should open a new chapter in the management and diagnosis of biliary tract diseases.

REFERENCES

1) Classen, M. and Safrany, L.: Endoscopic papillotomy and removal of gallstones. Brit. Med. J. 4: 371-374, 1975.
2) Classen, M. and Ossenberg, F.W.: Non-surgical removal of common bile duct stones. Gut 18: 760-769, 1977.
3) Cotton, P.B., Chapman, M., Whiteside, C.G., and Le Quesne, P.: Duodenoscopic papillotomy and gallstone removal. Brit. J. Surg. 63: 709-714, 1976.
4) Demling, L. and Classen, M. (eds.) Endoscopic Sphincterotomy of the Papilla of Vater. International Workshop Munich. Georg Thieme Verlag, Stuttgart, 1978.
5) Kawai, K., Akasaka, Y., Murakami, K., Tada, M., Kohli, Y., and Nakajima, M.: Endoscopic sphincterotomy of the ampulla of Vater. Gastrointest. Endosc. 20: 148-151, 1974.
6) Nakajima, M., Kimoto, K., Ikehara, H., Fukumoto, K., and Kawai, K.: Endoscopic sphincterotomy of the ampulla of Vater and removal of common duct stones. Am. J. Gastroenterol. 64: 34-43, 1975.
7) Nakajima, M., Akasaka, Y., Yamaguchi, K., Fujimoto, S., and Kawai, K.: Direct endoscopic visualization of the bile and pancreatic duct systems by peroral cholangiopancreatoscopy (PCPS). Gastrointest. Endosc. 24: 141-145, 1978.

 8) Nakajima, M., Akasaka, Y., and Kawai, K.: Endoscopic sphincterotomy (EST) of the papilla of Vater: Its techniques, significance and evaluation. In: Takemoto, T. and Kasugai, T. (eds.) Endoscopic Retrograde Cholangiopancreatography, pp. 73-93, Igaku-Shoin, Tokyo, 1979.

 9) Nakajima, M., Kizu, M., Akasaka, Y., and Kawai, K.: Five years experiences of endoscopic sphincterotomy in Japan: A collective study from 25 centers. Endoscopy 11: 138-141, 1979.

10) Nakajima, M., Kizu, M., Akasaka, Y., and Kawai, K.: Peroral cholangioscopy (PCS) under sliding tube guidance: A preliminary report of the instruments and techniques. In: Classen, M., Geenen, J., and Kawai, K. (eds.) International Workshop: The Papilla of Vater and Its Diseases, pp. 99-102, Gerhard Witzstrock, Baden-Baden, 1979.

11) Nakajima, M., Akasaka, Y., Yamaguchi, K., Kimoto, K., Fujimoto, S., Mitsuyoshi, Y., and Kawai, K.: Peroral cholangioscopy (PCS) and transendoscopic instrumentation of the biliary tract. Endoscopy. (in press)

12) Safrany, L.: Duodenoscopic sphincterotomy and gallstone removal. Gastroenterology 72: 338-343, 1977.

13) Safrany, L.: Endoscopic treatment of biliary-tract diseases. An international study. Lancet No. 4, 983-985, 1978.

14) Zimmon, D.S., Falkenstein, D.B., and Kessler, R.E.: Management of biliary calculi by endoscopic instrumentation (lithocenosis). Gastrointest. Endosc. 23: 82-86, 1976.

Case 1   Spontaneous passage of biliary stones after EST

A 68-year-old male. *Chief complaint:* epigastric pain with fever and jaundice.

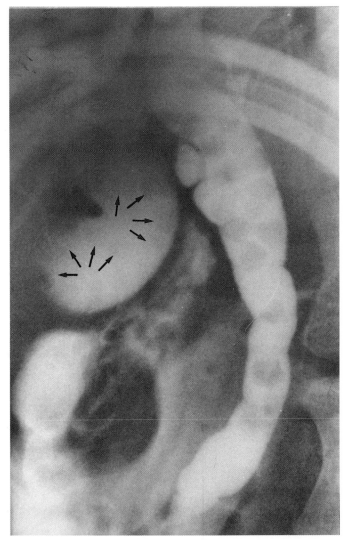

A. Endoscopic retrograde cholangiogram shows numerous stones within the common bile duct and several (arrows) within the gallbladder. Because the patient also had severe cardiac failure and was judged unfit for laparotomy, EST was attempted to relieve the debilitating cholestasis and sepsis due to biliary tract obstruction.

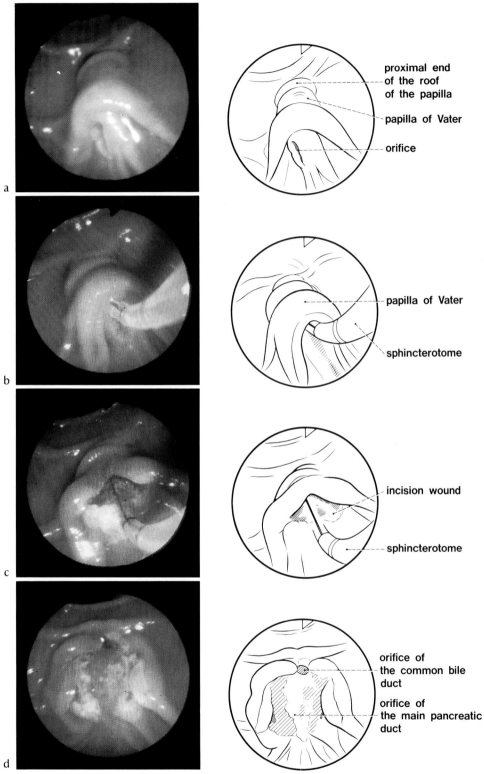

B. Endoscopic pictures of the papilla of Vater at EST (a, before sphincterotomy; b, sphinctero-tome in place; c, during the procedure; d, immediately following EST). After the EST, de-hydrocholic acid and cholecystokinin were given in the hope of facilitating a spontaneous passage of these stones.

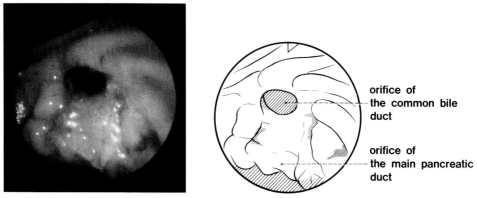

orifice of
the common bile
duct

orifice of
the main pancreatic
duct

C. Papilla of Vater one week after EST. An enlarged orifice of the distal common bile duct is seen at the deformed papilla.

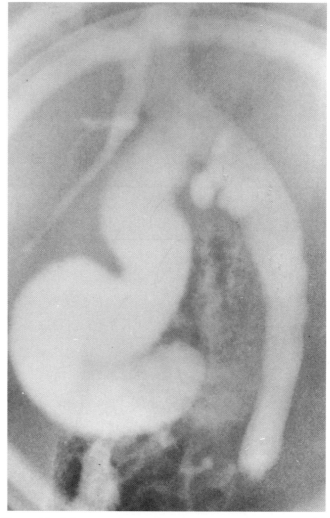

D. Repeat ERCP at this follow-up observation demonstrates no stones within the bile duct, indicating that all of the stones within the gallbladder as well as within the common bile duct have passed spontaneously through the incised papilla.

Case 2 Basket retrieval of a biliary tract stone after EST

A 54-year-old female. *Chief complaint:* right-upper quadrant pain with or without fever and probable jaundice. The patient had a laparotomy three years prior to this admission for gallstone disease.

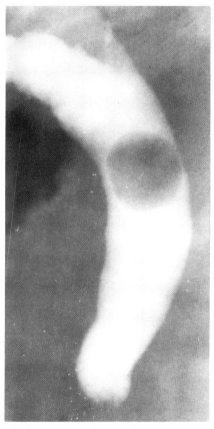

A. Endoscopic retrograde cholangiogram shows one residual or recurrent stone within the dilated common bile duct. As the patient did not want a repeat laparotomy, EST was required to remove the stone.

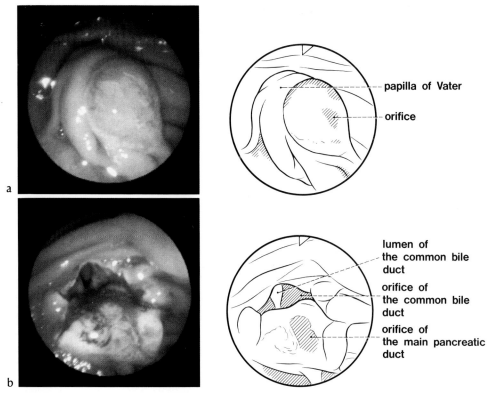

B. Endoscopic pictures of the papilla of Vater at EST. a, before sphincterotomy; b, immediately following the procedure.

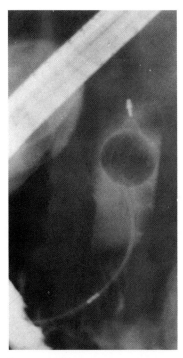

C. Immediately following the EST, a basket-tipped catheter passed through an endoscope was inserted into the common bile duct through the incised papilla and successfully caught and ensnared the stone under fluoroscopic control.

217

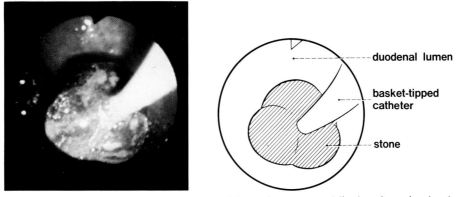

D. Endoscopic picture of the stone just extracted from the common bile duct into the duodenum through the incised papilla.

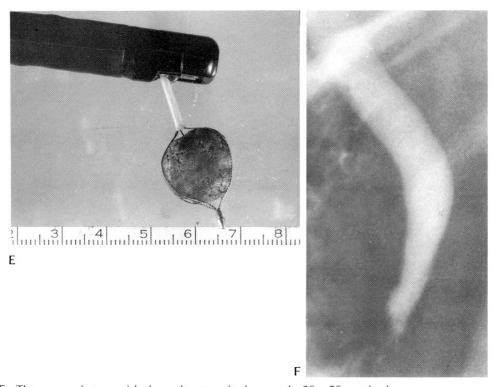

E

F

E. The removed stone with the endoscope via the mouth, 20 x 20 mm in size.
F. Repeat endoscopic retrograde cholangiogram demonstrates no stones within the biliary tract.

Case 3   Small polypoid carcinoma of the common bile duct

A 67-year-old female.   *Chief complaint:* abdominal pain with jaundice.   The patient had undergone a cholecystectomy for gallstone disease ten years previously.

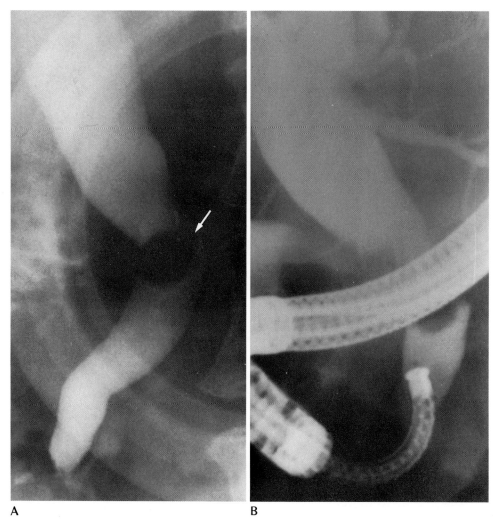

A   B

A. Endoscopic retrograde cholangiogram illustrates a round stone-like shadow within the common bile duct (arrow). This radiolucent shadow, however, did not move by varying the patient's position or by compressing the duct, suggesting the presence of a small polypoid tumor, not a stone, within the common bile duct.

B. X-ray picture shows the procedure of peroral cholangioscopy under sliding tube guidance after EST, which should give a further precise diagnosis of this interesting lesion. The tip of the cholangioscope introduced into the duct is confronting the tumorous lesion of the common bile duct.

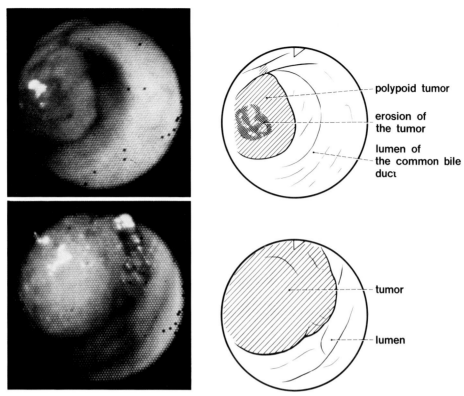

C. Cholangioscopic pictures of the tumor of the common bile duct. A reddish polypoid tumor is clearly seen within the ductal lumen. Biopsy specimen taken under direct vision at this procedure indicated a malignant development of the tumor.

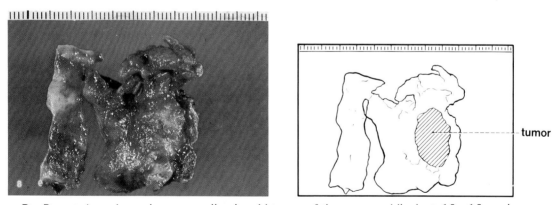

D. Resected specimen shows a small polypoid tumor of the common bile duct, 15 x 15 mm in size. No malignant invasion or metastases were found in the neighboring organs and regional lymph nodes at operation.

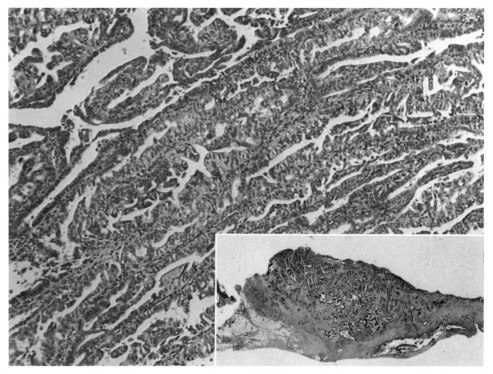

E. Photomicrograph of the tumor reveals a well-differentiated adenocarcinoma limited to the subserosal layer of the common bile duct wall.

7

Endoscopy of the Small Intestine

KAZUEI OGOSHI, M.D.

Based on clinical experience with duodenofiberscopy and colonoscopy, attempts at small intestinal observation have been reported by several endoscopists. Because of the length and tortuosity of the small bowel, many different types of fiberscopes have been developed for the observation of the jejunum and ileum.

In 1972, Hiratsuka reported the method of using a guide wire, previously placed through the digestive tract, to observe the entire small bowel. Soon afterward, Classen et al. also reported the advancement of a scope to the terminal ileum using the same method which Hiratsuka had described. This technique required from two to several days, because of the time needed for the guide wire to traverse the digestive tract. In addition, the biopsy channel was occupied by the gide wire, so a biopsy could not be done unless an enteroscope with two operating channels was used.

At about the same time, we succeeded in advancing a scope beyond the duodeno-jejunal flexure perorally without a guide wire. The small intestinal fiberscope used in our series has a large biopsy channel and employs a suction biopsy tube to obtain biopsy specimens from the proximal jejunum for the diagnosis of diffuse small bowel disease. Forceps biopsy is also obtained for the diagnosis of localized disease. This peroral small intestinal fiberscope technique is easy to perform and allows discovery of mucosal atrophy, diffuse disease and localized ulcers or tumors in the upper jejunum. On the other hand, we can not reach the ileum with this method, therefore, a second scope which is flexible, smaller in diameter and longer is being developed.

Equipment

The small intestinal fiberscope (Olympus SIF) is basically identical to the duodeno-fiberscope (Olympus JF), but is forward-viewing. Several kinds with different lengths have been devised and used. The Olympus SIF has the following specifications (Table 7-1).

An important advantage of the SIF scope is the provision of a suction biopsy tube which is similar to the Rubin tube. A 100 ml syringe is used to produce the vacuum which is registered on a meter and is then transmitted down the biopsy tube. This vacuum draws mucosa into the biopsy port (Figs. 7-1 and 7-2). For target biopsies, a biopsy forceps is available for use through this scope.

Preparation

Special patient preparation is not required. An anticholinergic and diazepam are injected intravenously as premedication just prior to the procedure.

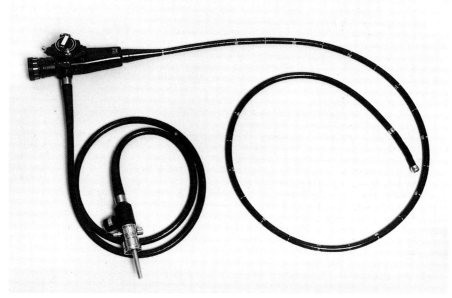

Fig. 7-1 Small intestinal fiberscope (Olympus SIF).

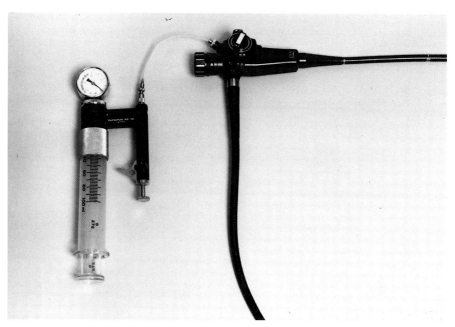

Fig. 7-2 Manipulated portion of the suction biopsy tube.

The contraindications for small intestinal fiberscopy are the same as those for gastroscopy or duodenoscopy. Because this scope can be advanced as far as 100 cm beyond the duodenojejunal flexure, the indications for peroral enteroscopy are limited to diffuse mucosal diseases or localized lesions of the upper jejunum.

During the examination, fluoroscopy is necessary to check the position of the scope.

As this scope has a bright illumination system and a good image fiber, no special light source is necessary.

Table 7-1 Specifications of the Olympus small intestinal fiberscope (SIF).

Range of observation	5 mm to 45 mm
Angle of view field	forward view 74°
Focusing	fixed focus
Diameter of distal end	10 mm
Bending angle	up 150°, down 120°
	right 90°, left 90°
Total length	1,770 mm (2,500 mm)
Working length	1,620 mm (2,350 mm)
Diameter of biopsy channel	2.8 mm
Diameter of suction biopsy tube	2.4 mm

Examination Technique

The method for advancing the scope to the second portion of the duodenum is the same as that for gastroduodenoscopy employing a forward-viewing scope.

The small field of view, flexibility and length of the scope make it more difficult to find the pylorus than in other types of upper GI endoscopy. In addition, the tip of the scope will easily U-turn in the stomach. For this reason, while in the stomach, the scope is advanced slowly and carefully, keeping the pyloric region in view. After inserting the scope through the pyloric ring, the descending duodenum will appear in the field of view. In some cases, beyond the pyloric ring as the scope is being advanced slowly with a full field of view, the tip of the scope must be withdrawn and returned to the stomach because of irregular bending or loop formation of the scope in the stomach. To avoid this condition, the scope is twisted until a regular counterclockwise loop is formed within the stomach. This technique is the same as that for loop formation in the sigmoid colon in colonoscopy. After this loop is formed, the scope is advanced smoothly to the third portion of the duodenum (Fig. 7-3).

When the tip of the scope reaches the duodenojejunal flexure, we have found the field of view is sometimes lost because the tip of the scope has pressed against the mucosal surface. In this situation, a full visual field may be required by effectively using the angulation wheels.

The most difficult part in advancing the scope to the jejunum is to pass the scope through the duodenojejunal flexure. In nearly 20 percent of cases, the scope was easily advanced downward from the duodenojejunal flexure. While in the other 80 percent of cases, the tip of the scope was advanced forming a counterclockwise loop beyond the duodenojejunal flexure. This facilitated natural and easy further advance of the scope in these cases.

After passing the duodenojejunal flexure, the tip of the scope will reach the jejunal mucosa. In the majority of cases, the scope was advanced until two and half loops formed beyond the duodenojejunal flexure. This length is about 100 cm beyond the duodenojejunal flexure (Fig. 7-4).

Finally fluoroscopic observation is necessary to confirm the position of the tip of the scope.

Endoscopic views of the jejunal mucosa at the original magnification are clear enough for clinical diagnosis. A glossy surface and sharp regular Kerckling folds are observed in the normal jejunum (Fig. 7-5).

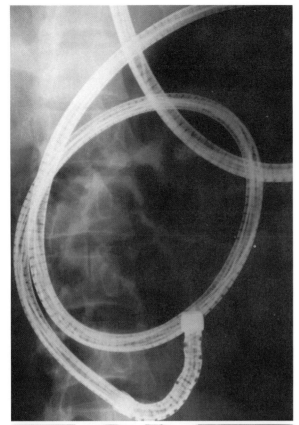

Fig. 7-3 The tip of the scope is advanced into the jejunum while a counterclockwise loop is formed in the stomach.

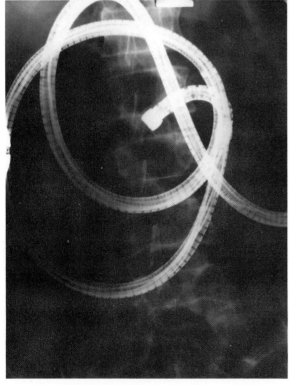

Fig. 7-4 The scope is inserted deeply beyond the duodenojejunal flexure.

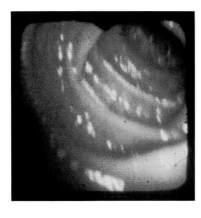

Fig. 7-5 Endoscopic picture of the jejunum. A glossy surface and sharp regular Kerckling folds are observed.

Biopsy Technique

For taking an intestinal biopsy through the SIF scope, both biopsy forceps and a suction biopsy tube are available. The advantage of the suction biopsy obtained through the SIF scope is that the biopsy material is larger, undamaged and better suited for diagnosis. On the other hand, the ability to take a target biopsy in this manner is inferior to that of the biopsy forceps method.

After a suitable area for biopsy has been selected, the suction biopsy tube, in which the mechanism has previously been set, is advanced until the tip of the biopsy tube appears in the field of view.

A red spot which lies opposite the biopsy port at the tip of the tube indicates the spot where the suction port is pressed against the jejunal mucosa to obtain a biopsy. Vacuum pressure is applied by drawing the plunger of the syringe. The meter should register about 50 cm of mercury. The mucosa is then drawn into the biopsy port in one or two seconds and cut by releasing the biopsy trigger. The biopsy tube is with-drawn immediately.

Specimens taken by the suction tube measure about 2 x 3 cm in mean size and are 3 mg in wet weight. The shape of the villi is clearly demonstrated. Such specimens are easy to cut tangentially, making it possible to measure the height and diameter of villi and secretory glands (Fig. 7-6).

A small red spot or slight hemorrhage indicates that a biopsy specimen has been taken (Fig. 7-7). Multiple biopsies are obtainable in a short period of time.

Results and Discussion

Small intestinal fiberscopy with an SIF scope was successfully performed in 122 cases. Of these, there were two cases with protein-losing enteropathy in which biopsy specimens revealed marked dilatation of lymph vessels in the jejunal mucosa. Two cases of localized jejunal disease were also observed; one with a leiomyosarcoma and one with nonspecific ulceration in the jejunum.

As already mentioned, several kinds of instruments for enteroscopy have been developed independently but are not yet standardized because it is impossible to accurately examine the entire intestine with one type of scope.

Although small intestinal disease is relatively rare, many techniques now exist to evaluate it. A short segment of the terminal ileum, in which intestinal disease is often observed, can be examined by passing a colonoscope through the ileocecal valve. To

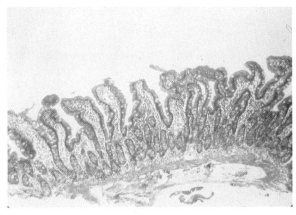

Fig. 7-6 Biopsy specimen taken through the biopsy tube.

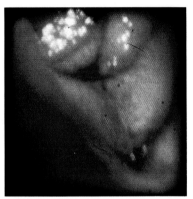

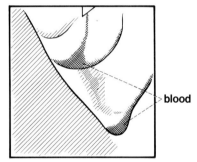

blood

Fig. 7-7 After mucosal biopsy by the suction tube, a small red spot indicates the place where a biopsy specimen has been taken.

observe the entire small intestine, the method of using a guide wire can be employed. A peroral small intestinal fiberscope is useful for examining diffuse intestinal disease of the upper part of the jejunum but it is impossible to examine deeper portion of the small intestine with it.

Recently, a new type of long and floppy fiberscope which passes down the small intestine spontaneously has been used experimentally (Figs. 7-8 and 7-9).

An ideal fiberscope which has a large biopsy channel and can be passed down the entire small intestine is desired. Once designed, the technique could be standardized and used for diagnosing all types of intestinal disease, thereby replacing the many different methods used today.

REFERENCES

1) Classen, M., Frühmorgen, P., Koch, H., and Demling, L.: Enteroskopie: Fiberendoskopie von Jejunum und Ileum. Dtsch. Med. Wschr. 11: 409-411, 1972.
2) Classen, M., Frühmorgen, P., Koch, H., and Demling, L.: Enteroscopy: Peroral and peranal endoscopy of the small bowel. In: Demling, L. and Classen, M. (eds.) Endoscopy of the Small Intestine with Retrograde Pancreato-Cholangiography, pp. 113-120, Georg Thieme Verlag, Stuttgart, 1973.

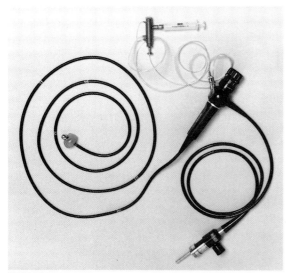

Fig. 7-8 A new sonde type of small intestinal fiberscope.

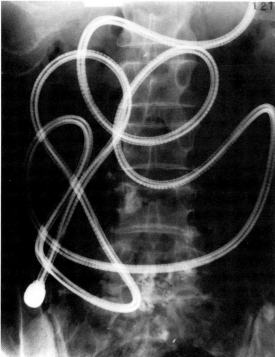

Fig. 7-9 A sonde type of scope is inserted deeply into the small intestine.

3) Hiratsuka, H.: Enteroscopy and biopsy of the small intestine. In: Demling, L. and Classen, M. (eds.) Endoscopy of the Small Intestine with Retrograde Pancreato-Cholangiography, pp. 108-112, Georg Thieme Verlag, Stuttgart, 1973.
4) Ogoshi, K. and Hara, Y.: Clinical application of the small intestinal fiberscope (Olympus). In: Demling, L. and Classen, M. (eds.) Endoscopy of the Small Intestine with Retrograde Pancreato-Cholangiography, pp. 120-123, Georg Thieme Verlag, Stuttgart, 1973.
5) Ogoshi, K., Hara, Y., and Ashizawa, S.: New technic for small intestinal fiberscopy. Gastrointest. Endoscopy 20: 64-65, 1973.
6) Salmon, P.: Fibre-Optic Endoscopy. Pitman Medical, London, 1974. pp. 128-138.

Case 1   Normal mucosa of the small intestine

A 60-year-old male. *Chief complaint:* diarrhea. *Final diagnosis:* irritable colon.

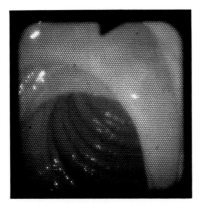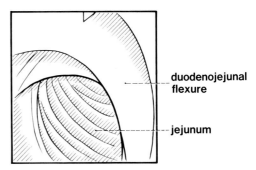

A. Normal endoscopic view of the duodenojejunal flexure. At the duodenojejunal flexure, a sharp angulation which may prevent smooth insertion of the scope, appears in the view field.

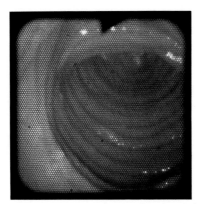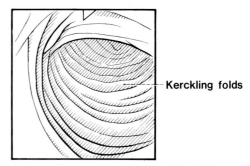

B. Normal mucosa beyond the duodenojejunal flexure. Beyond the duodenojejunal flexure, a glossy surface and sharp and regular Kerckling folds are observed.

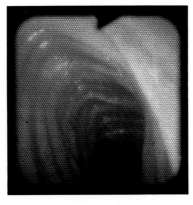

C. Normal jejunal mucosa. The tip of the scope can be reached about 100 cm beyond the duodenojejunal flexure. Jejunal mucosa is clearly observed.

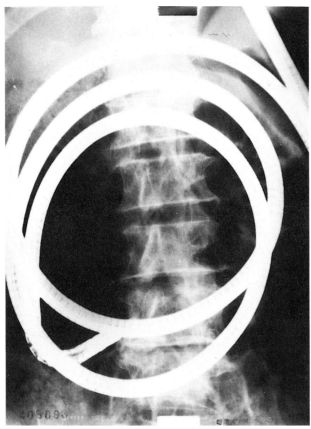

D. SIF is deeply inserted into the jejunum. At present, about 100 cm is considered maximum length for jejunal observation.

Case 2   **Leiomyosarcoma of the jejunum**

A 38-year-old male. *Chief complaints:* Abdominal pain and a palpable tumor. *Present illness:* The patient was admitted on October 13, 1976 for abdominal pain of several months' duration. There was a firm mass about 8 x 7 cm in size with slight tenderness in the left upper quadrant. Laboratory data on admission revealed acute inflammation and positive occult blood in the stool. Routine upper GI series, gastroduodenoscopy, hepatic scintigraphy, barium enema and ERCP gave no positive findings.

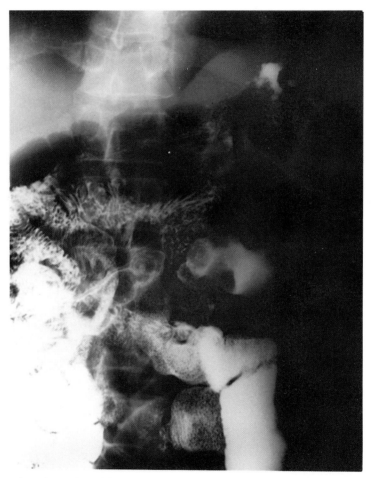

A. Small bowel radiography with double contrast method shows a small barium fleck in the proximal portion of the jejunum.

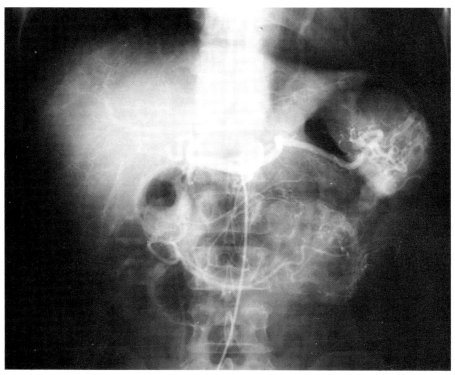

B. Superior mesentric arteriogram. A large number of vessels (arrows) supplied by jejunal arteries are observed in the tumor. The middle colic artery is displaced downward by the mass. A well-defined tumor shadow is observed in the venous phase.

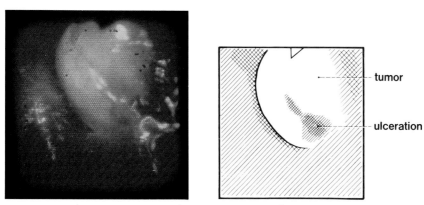

C. Small intestinal fiberscopic finding (with Olympus SIF). A protruding lesion like a submucosal tumor with central ulceration is observed at the upper part of the jejunum.

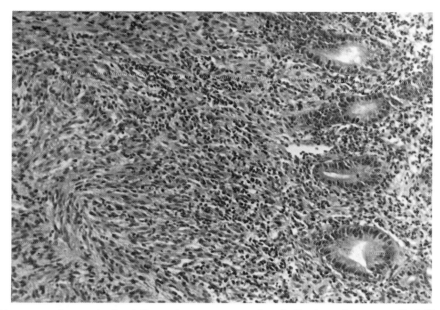

D. Biopsy specimen obtained from the tumor reveals spindle-shaped tumor cells infiltrating into the jejunal mucosa from the submucosal layer. H.E., x 100

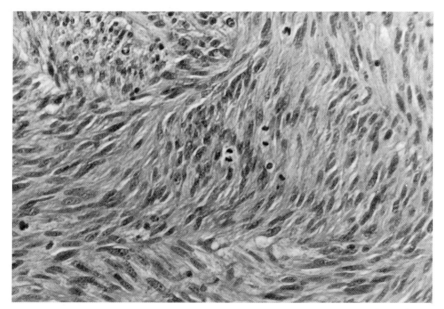

E. A mass measuring about 7.5 x 6 x 5 cm with a central cavity was resected from the proximal part of the jejunum (about 5 cm from the duodenojejunal flexure) and revealed a leiomyosarcoma histologically. H.E., x 200

8

Endoscopy of the Large Intestine

SEIBI KOBAYASHI, M.D.

Preparation of the Patient

First of all, adequate cleaning of the colon and rectum is very important for a successful examination. The patient is required to take a low residue diet for two to three days before the examination. A mild laxative, 20 g of magnesium sulphate, is given the evening before the day of the examination and the patient is fasted overnight. Two enemas of 1 quart of tap water each are given two hours and one hour before the examination. Just prior to the examination, the patient is injected with 20 mg of hyoscine N-butylbromide (Buscopan) intravenously or intramuscularly to sedate intestinal motility. Five to 10 mg of intravenous diazepam may be given to apprehensive patients.

Preparation of the Instrument

Prepare the instrument according to the manufacturer's directions. Photograph the patient's name through the scope so that the subsequent pictures will be properly identified. Make sure the controls, air insufflation, water, suction, etc. are working properly before instrumentation. The author employs the Olympus instruments CF-MB3, CF-MB3R, CF-LB3 and TCF-1S (Fig. 8-1).

Technique

At the beginning of colonoscopy, the patient is required to lie in the supine position on the endoscopy table and a digital examination is performed to check the rectum and lubricate the anal region with Xylocaine jelly.

The colonofiberscope is introduced into the rectum under the guidance of the right index finger with the patient lying in the left lateral decubitus position. After the scope passes through the rectosigmoid junction, the so-called "slide-by" technique is employed and as long as the mucosa with blood vessels is seen to "slide-by", it is usually safe to continue advancing. If the mucosa does not "slide-by", further instrumentation with this technique should be abandoned and the scope should be withdrawn to visualize the lumen. Further insertion can then be attempted under direct vision.

The patient is required to turn onto the back after the instrument has reached approximately 30 to 50 cm from the anus. In this position, the sigmoid and descending colon are more extended to facilitate further advancement of the scope. The instrument can be introduced up to the splenic flexure or somewhere in the descending colon in most cases without fluoroscopic control (Fig. 8-2).

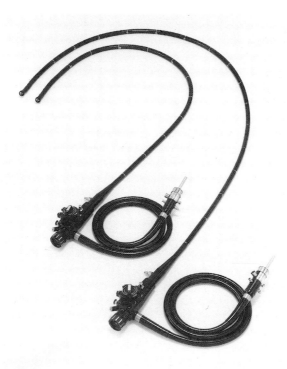

Fig. 8-1 Olympus colonofiberscopes CF-MB3 (left) and CF-LB3 (right).

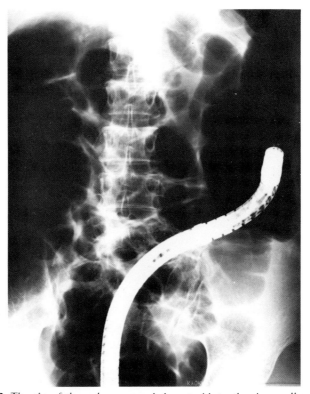

Fig. 8-2 The tip of the colonoscope is inserted into the descending colon.

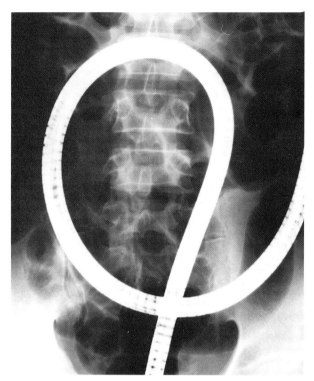

Fig. 8-3 So-called "alpha maneuver".

In order to examine beyond the splenic flexure, a long colonoscope is employed usually under fluoroscopic control. After the tip of the colonoscope has reached deep into the sigmoid colon, the so-called "alpha maneuver" is occasionally attempted by having an assistant rotate the tube of the scope in a counterclockwise direction (Fig. 8-3). At that time, the right lateral position of the patient is usually very helpful to bring the sigmoid colon easily on the right side of the abdominal cavity. The patient is now turned on the back and the scope is advanced through the sigmoid, crossing the right lower quadrant across the midline of the abdomen and up the descending colon. Reaching the splenic flexure, the tip of the scope is hooked tightly in the end of the transverse colon and straightening of the tube of the instrument is done by turning the tube in a clockwise direction with simultaneous withdrawal of the tube. A plastic sliding tube placed over the instrument prior to examination is then slowly inserted over the instrument up to the lower descending colon to maintain the straightening of the sigmoid and descending colon during examination.

Some experts do this maneuver without fluoroscopic control, but the author recommends use of fluoroscopy to make the proper position of the tip of the scope certain, thereby facilitating the advance of the scope to the transverse, the ascending colon and the cecum with relative ease. Passage of the instrument through the transverse colon may be difficult because the tube extends deep into the lesser pelvis on many occasions. Once the instrument reaches the hepatic flexure, an attempt should be made to straighten the transverse colon by withdrawing the instrument (Fig. 8-4). The instrument is then easily advanced to the cecum through the ascending colon. Visualization of the entire colon is best achieved while the instrument is being withdrawn. Redun-

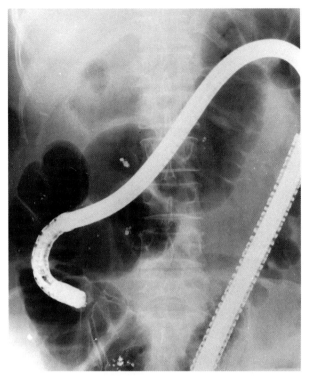

Fig. 8-4 An attempt should be made to straighten the transverse colon to make further instrumentation easy.

dant transverse colon may permit an unusual way of instrumentation into the cecum on occasions (Fig. 8-5). Biopsy and brushing cytology can also be taken under direct vision (Fig. 8-6).

The role of the assistant is very important in order to perform the examination skillfully. While the operator manipulates the buttons for air, water and suction and the angle controls, the assistant can advance or withdraw the instrument according to the operator's directions. A teaching attachment can help the assistant do the work more efficiently and be especially valuable to the operator.

Indications and Contraindications

Indications

Indications for colonoscopy are as follows:

    A. Diagnostic colonoscopy
        1. Abnormal barium enema
        2. Abnormal sigmoidoscopy
        3. Unexplained colonic symptoms
        4. Lower gastrointestinal bleeding
        5. Evaluation of postoperative colon
        6. Assessment of inflammatory bowel disease in selected cases
    B. Therapeutic colonoscopy
        1. Polypectomy
        2. Removal of foreign body

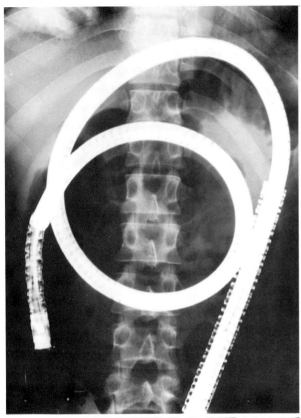

Fig. 8-5 An unusual way of instrumentation into the cecum because of redundant transverse colon.

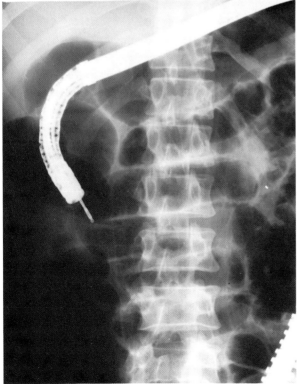

Fig. 8-6 Biopsy and brush cytology can be taken under direct vision.

Contraindications

Colonoscopy is contraindicated under the following circumstances.

- A. Fulminant ulcerative colitis
- B. Fulminant granulomatous colitis
- C. Acute diverticulitis
- D. Severe ischemic bowel disease
- E. Acute severe irradiation colitis
- F. Peritonitis
- G. Pregnancy

Complications

Bleeding and perforation are two major complications of colonoscopy and procto-sigmoidoscopy. Of nearly 3,000 colonoscopic examinations in our own series, bleeding was encountered in only one instance due to rupture of a hemorrhoidal vein by instru-mentation.

The complications can be avoided by cautious performance of the examination.

Table 8-1 summarizes the complications of bleeding and perforation, respectively, in 3,850 colonoscopies and 901 polypectomies reported in Gastroenterology by Berci et al.

Table 8-1 Complications *.

Colonoscopy	3,850
Polypectomy	901
Bleeding	
Immediate	4
Delayed	2
Mortality	0
Perforation	10
Diagnosed immediately	7
Diagnosed late	3
Related to manipulation	7
Related to coagulation	3
Mortality	1

* From Berci, G. et al.: Complications of colono-scopy and polypectomy. Report of the Southern California Society for Gastrointestinal Endoscopy. Gastroenterology 67: 584-585, 1974.

They concluded that the morbidity of colonoscopy and colonoscopic polypectomy compares quite favorably with the 20.0 percent rate reported in patients undergoing laparotomy, colotomy, and polypectomy.

Proctosigmoidoscopy is a much safer procedure in experienced hands; only 4 severe injuries were recorded in 350,000 examinations according to Jackman.

Another report of Geenen's described that the incidence of major complications reported from specialized centers has ranged from 0.1 to 1.9 percent.

Colonoscopic Polypectomy

Polypectomy under colonoscopic observation has become feasible anywhere in the colon and rectum. The polyps for endoscopic polypectomy are usually pedunculated or semipedunculated. Blood type and bleeding tendency are investigated beforehand, for there are always risks of perforation and bleeding.

For performing a polypectomy, some additional equipments are needed, for example, electrosurgical snare, power source for snare, carbon dioxide source, etc. Just prior to polypectomy, all of the equipments should be checked to see if they are working properly.

Bowel preparation for polypectomy is more vigorous than for routine colonoscopy, in order to remove the explosive gases, hydrogen and methane. Preparation for routine colonoscopy mentioned earlier is usually enough to remove the gases. However, the use of carbon dioxide completely obviates the possibility of explosion.

With the technique of colonoscopy previously described, polyps are visualized at any point in the colon and rectum. A polypectomy snare is passed through the biopsy channel of the colonoscope and then is advanced to make a loop. After the loop is passed over the body of the polyp, the snare wire is positioned at the stalk of the polyp and tightened around the stalk. A slowly increasing coagulation current is applied from a diathermy power source of the Olympus PSD until local coagulation is visible and subsequent cutting is made. The removed polyp is sucked into the tip of the colonoscope which is then withdrawn from the rectum. After removal of the polyp, the colonoscope is again inserted to inspect the polypectomy site and the maneuver is terminated after making certain that there is no serious complication at the site.

The largest world experience with endoscopic polypectomy for colonic polyps is at the Beth Israel Medical Center in New York, where over 2,000 polyps had been endoscopically removed until 1974 without a single death and with only one complication requiring operative intervention. Laparotomy is now reserved for polyps not suitable for endoscopic resection or where a question of residual cancer exists. Experience with endoscopic resection has called for : 1) re-assessment of colonic polyps in terms of their malignant potential and 2) clarification of the indications for laparotomy and bowel resection subsequent to or instead of endoscopic removal. Among all polypoid lesions 0.5 cm or greater in size in the Beth Israel series, a variety of pathologic types was encountered. If only the neoplastic polyps were considered, the incidence of "malignant change" was 10.5 percent for 855 polyps analyzed. Nearly 10 percent of "malignant change" was also noted in our own series of colonic polypectomy. There is, however, a need to clarify terminology and to differentiate between carcinoma in situ and invasive cancer whenever possible. Carcinoma in situ does not recur or metastasize and requires no treatment other than polyp removal. When "invasive" cancer is present (4.5% of neoplastic polyps) or the lesion is a "polypoid carcinoma" each case must be individually evaluated.

REFERENCES

1) Berci, G., Panish, J.F., Schapiro, M., and Corlin, R.: Complications of colonoscopy and polypectomy. Report of the Southern California Society for Gastrointestinal Endoscopy. Gastroenterology 67: 584-585, 1974.
2) Geenen, J.F., Schmitt, M.G., Jr., Wallace, C.W., and Hogan, W.J.: Major complications of colonoscopy. Bleeding and perforation. Am. J. Dis. 20: 231-235, 1970.

3) Jackman, R.J.: Rigid tube proctosigmoidoscopy. History, anatomy, indications, technic. In: Berry, L.H. (ed.) Gastrointestinal Pan-Endoscopy, pp. 439-460, Charles C Thomas, Springfield, Ill., 1974.

4) Kobayashi, S., Yoshii, Y., and Kasugai, T.: Fibercolonoscopy: Effective use in symptomatic patients with negative barium enema. Endoscopy 7: 63-67, 1975.

5) Overholt, B.F.: Flexible fiberoptic sigmoidoscopy. Technique and preliminary results. Cancer 28: 122-126, 1971.

6) Overholt, B.F.: Colonoscopy. A review. Gastroenterology 68: 1308, 1975.

7) Ragins, H., Shinya, H., and Wolff, W.I.: The explosive potential of colonic gas during colonoscopic electrosurgical polypectomy. Surg. Gynec. Obstet. 138: 554-556, 1974.

8) Rogers, B.H.G.: Instructions for colonoscopy. ACMI Instruction Manual, 1974.

9) Sakai, Y.: The technic of colonofiberscopy. Dis. Colon & Rectum 15: 403-412, 1972.

10) Shinya, H., Eddy, J.F., Jr., and Overholt, B.F.: Fiberoptic colonoscopy: History, anatomy, indication, technic and pathology. In: Berry, L.H. (ed.) Gastrointestinal Pan-Endoscopy, pp. 409-417, Charles C Thomas, Springfield, Ill., 1974.

11) Waye, J.D.: Colonoscopy: A clinical view. The Mount Sinai J. Med. 42: 1-34, 1975.

12) Wolff, W.I., and Shinya, H.: Endoscopic polypectomy. Therapeutic and clinicopathologic aspects. Cancer 36: 683-690, 1975.

Case 1 Normal colonic mucosa

A 45-year-old female. *Chief complaint:* constipation.

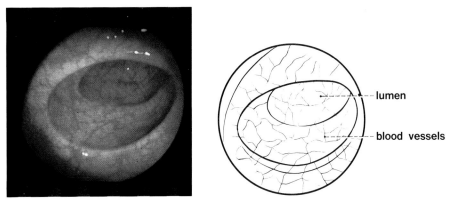

A. Normal sigmoid colon. The sigmoid colon is usually redundant, making a sharp angulation in many places and instrumentation difficult. Normal mucosa shows fine vascular patterns.

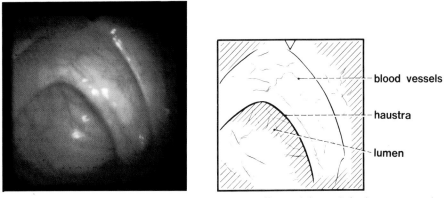

B. Normal transverse colon. The transverse colon is usually straight and the instrumentation is much easier than in the sigmoid colon. Normal mucosa shows fine vascular patterns with sharply round haustration.

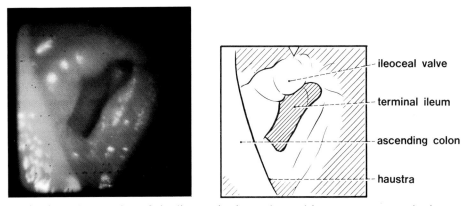

C. Ileocecal valve. An opening of the ileocecal valve and greenish contents are seen in the terminal ileum through the opening.

Case 2   Chronic ulcerative colitis : operated case for severe disease

A 32-year-old female. *Chief complaint:* bloody stools. A diagnosis of ulcerative colitis was made elsewhere one month prior to the first visit to the Aichi Cancer Center Hospital (ACCH).

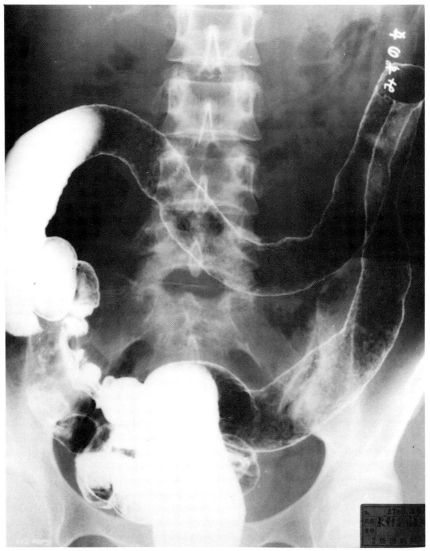

A. Barium enema shows no haustration and numerous ulcerations throughout the colon and rectum associated with dilatation of the terminal ileum. The diagnosis was chronic ulcerative colitis with backwash ileitis.

243

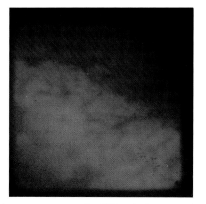
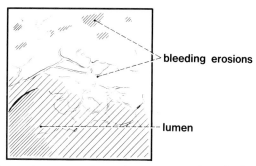

bleeding erosions

lumen

B. Colonoscopy reveals diffusely hyperemic and erosive mucosa from the rectum to the splenic flexure. The mucosa bled easily with instrumentation. Because of no improvement with medical treatment, the patient underwent total proctocolectomy with ileostomy.

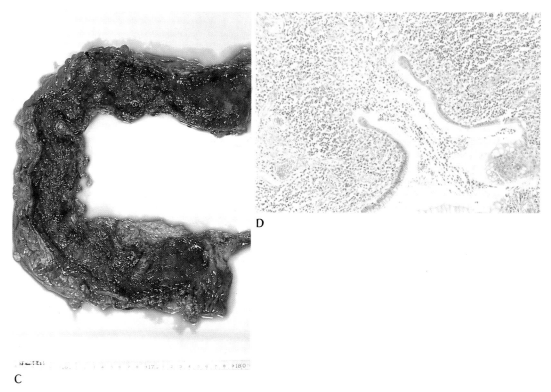

D

C

C. The gross specimen demonstrates pseudopolyposis and ulcerations throughout the large intestine.

D. Histological study shows a crypt abscess characteristic of chronic ulcerative colitis. H.E., x 100

Case 3   Chronic ulcerative colitis : chronic continuous type

A 65-year-old male. *Chief complaint:* bloody stools.   He first developed mucobloody stools one year ago, which have increased in severity.

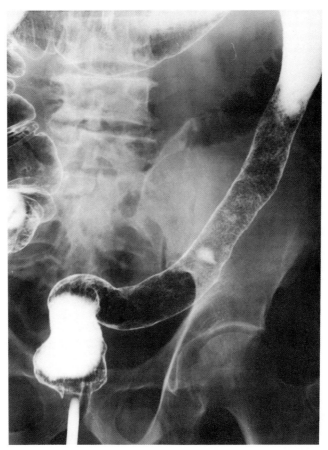

A. Barium enema reveals narrowing and shortening, no haustration of the sigmoid and descending colon with numerous ulcerations.   Radiological diagnosis was ulcerative colitis.

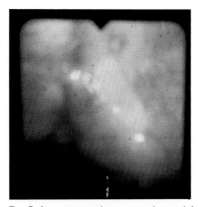 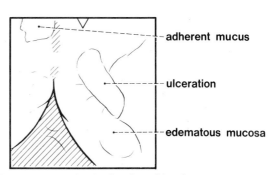

B. Colonoscopy shows an ulcer with edematous margins in the sigmoid colon.

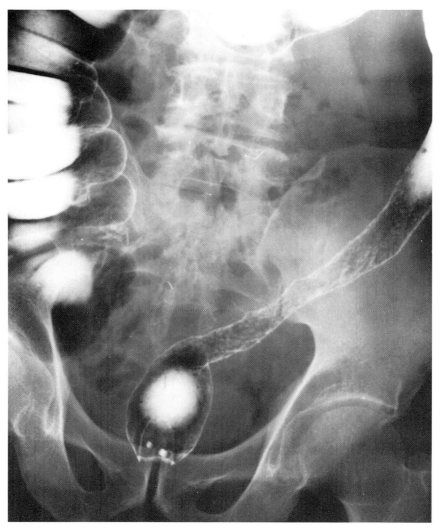

C. Barium enema one year later demonstrating more narrowing and shortening of the sigmoid colon with pseudopolyposis.

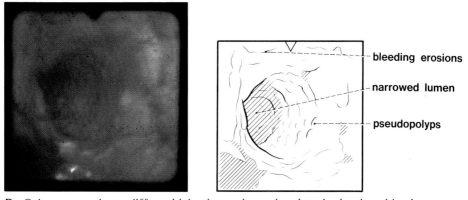

D. Colonoscopy shows diffuse thickening and pseudopolyps in the sigmoid colon.

Case 4   Chronic ulcerative colitis in remission : relapsing type

A 22-year-old male.   *Chief complaint:* mucobloody stools which started five months ago.

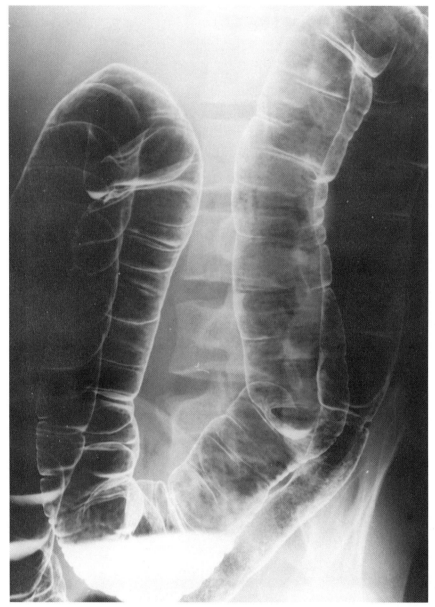

A. Barium enema reveals numerous small ulcerations diffusely from the rectum to the transverse colon, being consistent with the diagnosis of chronic ulcerative colitis.

Colonoscopy revealed a friable mucosa which easily bled by a touch with the instrument and vague appearance of small blood vessels in the rectum and the colon. Biopsy demonstrated severe active inflammation which was non-specific.

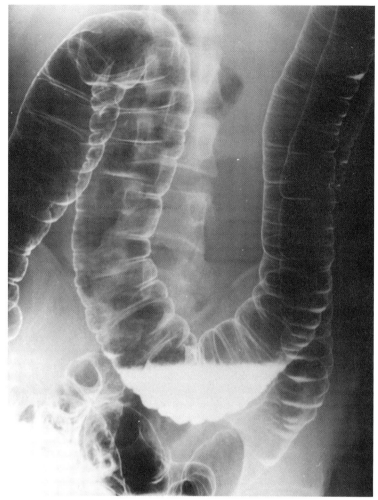

B. Barium enema three years later showing no evidence of ulcerations and appearance of haustration.

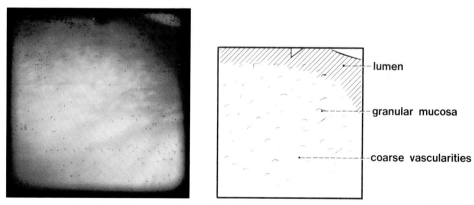

C. Colonoscopy at that time demonstrating yellowish patchy, finely granular mucosa with no ulceration and no vascular transparency, findings that indicated ulcerative colitis at the quiescent stage. No contact bleeding is noted.

Case 5   Crohn's colitis : operated case

A 21-year-old male. *Chief complaint:* diarrhea of three years' duration. Three years prior to this admission, he underwent an operation for a perianal abscess and afterwards had surgery for an anal fistula on several occasions.

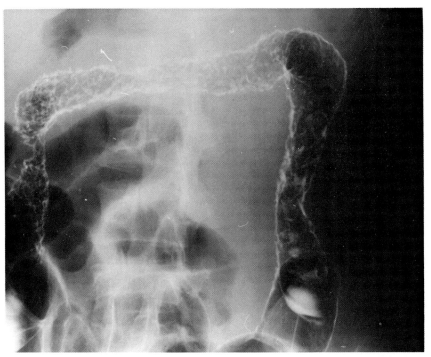

A. Barium enema reveals a coarsely nodular mucosal appearance abruptly from the mid-descending colon to the ascending colon. Crohn's colitis is suspected.

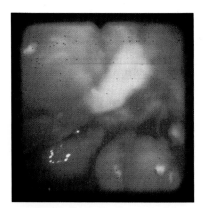
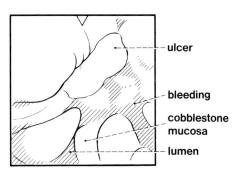

B. Colonoscopic observation is normal up to the mid-descending colon where a cobblestone-appearing mucosa starts with multiple longitudinal ulcers.
The diagnosis is most likely Crohn's disease of the colon. However, colonic tuberculosis is not entirely excluded. Colonoscopic biopsy demonstrated only non-specific chronic inflammation.

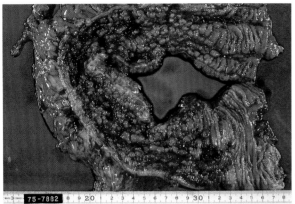

C. The resected specimen by a subtotal colectomy shows typical cobblestone mucosa with a number of longitudinal ulcers, characteristic of Crohn's disease.

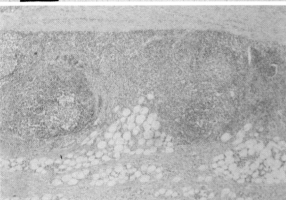

D. The pathological diagnosis is consistent with Crohn's disease involving the terminal ileum to the descending colon, because there is transmural inflammation with non-caseous granulomata. H.E., x 100

Case 6   Crohn's colitis : medically treated case

A 28-year-old male.   *Chief complaints:* right lower quadrant pain, high fever and an anal fistula.

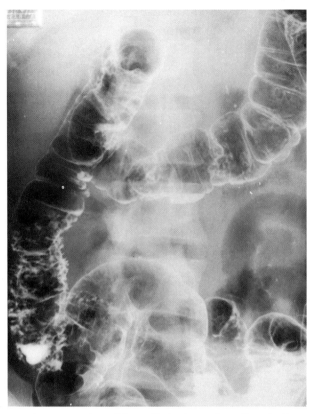

A. Barium enema reveals a narrowing with multiple deep ulcerations in the cecum and the proximal half of the ascending colon and some skip lesions in the hepatic flexure and transverse colon.
The diagnosis was most likely Crohn's disease with the findings of the terminal ileum shown on small intestinal follow-through series.

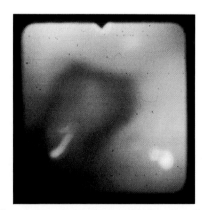
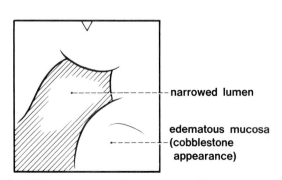

narrowed lumen

edematous mucosa
(cobblestone
appearance)

B. Colonoscopy shows large nodules, so-called "cobblestone mucosa", in the ascending colon.

251

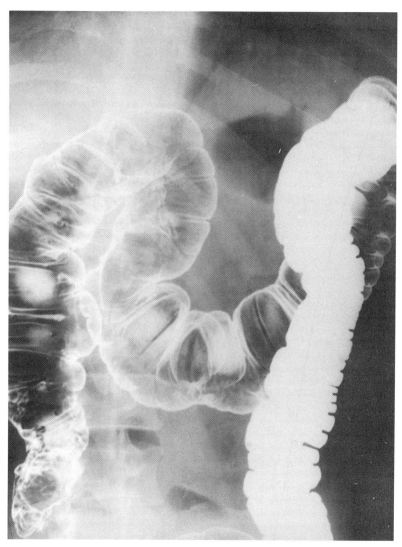

C. Barium enema. He had done well until approximately three years later when he developed high fever and severe right lower quadrant pain at which time this barium enema showed more narrowing with a cobblestone appearance in the ascending colon.

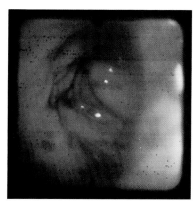 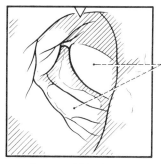

thickened mucosal folds in a narrowed lumen of the ascending colon

D. Colonoscopy at that time again revealing a cobblestone mucosa.

Case 7   Colonic tuberculosis

A 58-year-old male. *Chief complaint:* palpitation in the right lateral abdomen. Nearly 30 years ago during wartime, he had had colonic resection for tuberculosis of the ileocecal region.

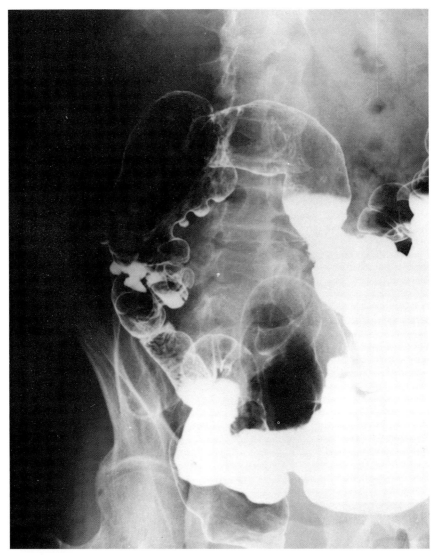

A. Barium enema shows a partial narrowing and multiple diverticula in the ascending colon and cecum with evidence of previous colonic surgery. The diagnostic impression is most likely tuberculosis of the colon.

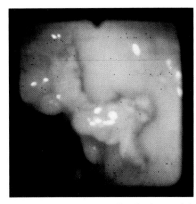 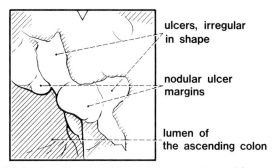

ulcers, irregular
in shape

nodular ulcer
margins

lumen of
the ascending colon

B. Colonoscopy visualizes the lesion with multiple diverticula and irregular ulcerations with whitish exudate in the ascending colon. The diagnostic impression is also tuberculosis of the colon.

Mantoux reaction was strongly positive. The patient was treated medically and is doing well. The latest barium enema showed significant improvement.

Case 8   Colonic polyp : sessile type

A 35-year-old female. *Chief complaint:* bloody stools. She developed rectal bleeding at which time barium enema revealed a polypoid lesion in the sigmoid colon, suspected of being early colonic cancer. Surgical polypectomy was performed and the histo-logical examination of the polypoid lesion demonstrated a well-differentiated adeno-carcinoma at the tip.

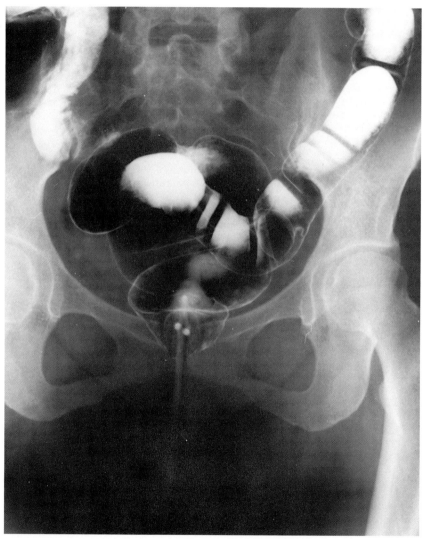

A. Follow-up barium enema several years later. A small polyp is seen in the sigmoid colon.

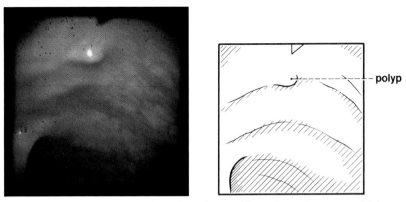

B. Colonoscopy also reveals a small sessile polyp at 40 cm from the anus, which was an adenomatous polyp in a biopsy specimen.

Case 9   Colonic polyp : pedunculated type

A 63-year-old male. *Chief complaint:* asymptomatic. He had a barium enema because both parents had died of rectal cancer.

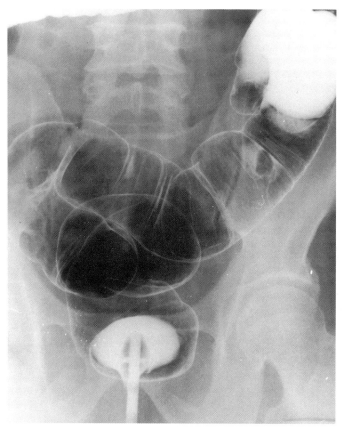

A. Barium enema reveals a pedunculated polyp in the sigmoid colon. The guaiac test for occult blood in the stools was negative.

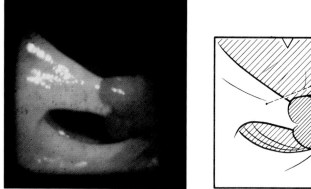
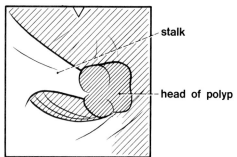

B. Colonoscopy demonstrates the pedunculated polyp 50 cm from the anus. Polypectomy was performed endoscopically on the same day.

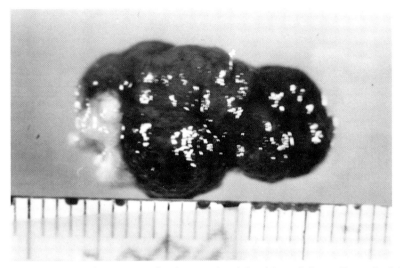

C. The gross specimen shows part of polyp on the right side and the stalk on the left side.

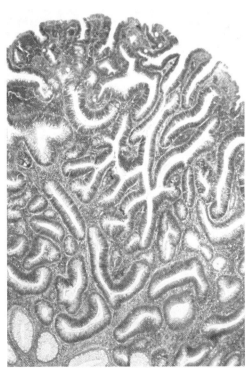

D. The histological examination demonstrates an adenoma with slight atypia. H.E., x 40

Case 10   Colonic polyp : polypectomy

A 47-year-old female. *Chief complaint:* bloody stools. She presented with rectal bleeding three years ago and was recommended for surgical resection of a colonic polyp detected on barium enema.

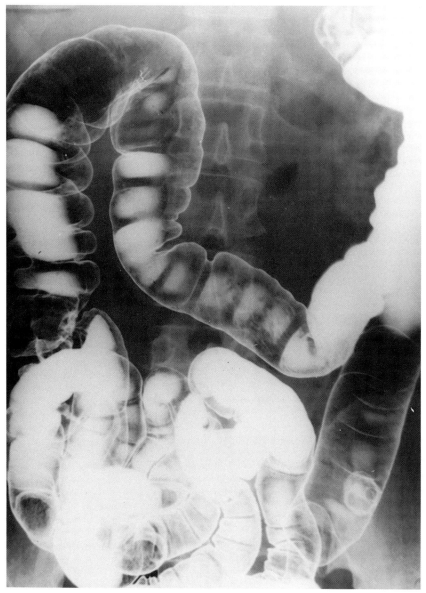

A. Barium enema reveals a polyp with a short stalk in the descending colon.

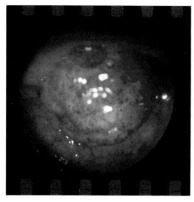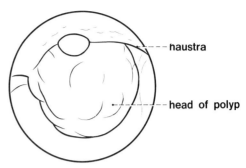

B. Colonoscopy visualizes the lesion 40 cm from the anus. Biopsy showed an adenomatous polyp with slight atypia and a polypectomy was done through the endoscope.

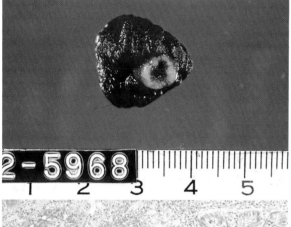

C. Colonoscopically resected polyp.

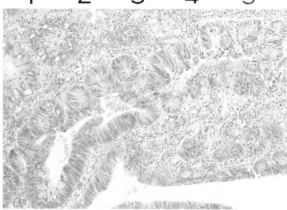

D. Histological examination demonstrates a border-line lesion with cellular and structural atypia. H.E., x 100

Case 11   Polypectomy for early colonic cancer

A 66-year-old male. *Chief complaint:* bloody stools. He presented with rectal bleeding four months ago.

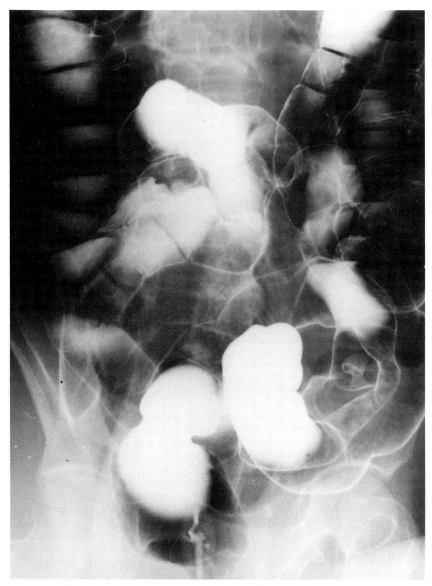

A. Barium enema reveals a pedunculated polyp in the sigmoid colon.

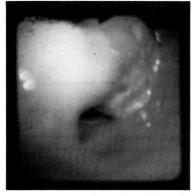
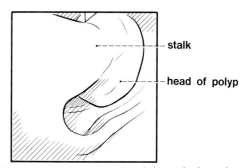

stalk

head of polyp

B. Colonoscopy reveals the polyp 35 cm from the anus and it was removed through the colonoscope at that time.

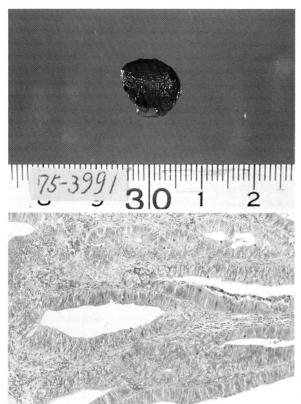

75-3991

C. The removed polyp is 13 x 12 x 9 mm in size.

D. The final histology demonstrates a well-differentiated adenocarcinoma in the polypoid structure, confined to the mucosa. H.E., x 100

Case 12   Cancer in adenoma

A 56-year-old male. *Chief complaint:* asymptomatic. He was further evaluated because of positive occult blood in the stools.

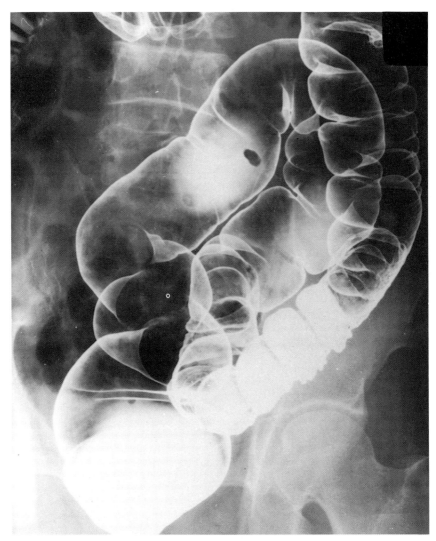

A. Barium enema reveals a polypoid lesion in the rectosigmoid colon.

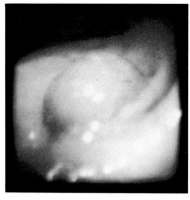
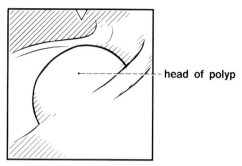

head of polyp

B. Colonoscopy reveals a semipedunculated polyp on the left posterior wall 20 cm from the anus. Biopsy demonstrated adenoma with severe atypia. Colonoscopic polypectomy was performed.

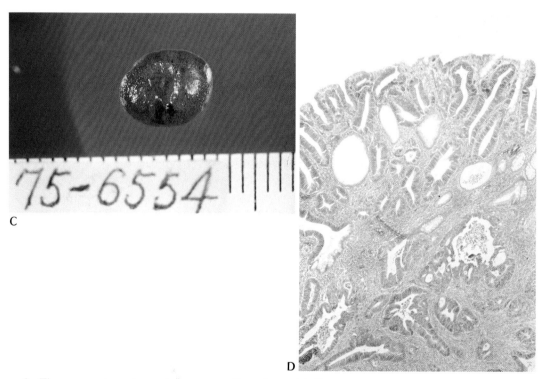

C

D

C. The removed specimen shows a smooth surface with fine textures.
D. The histological examination demonstrates malignant glands with desmoplastic stromal reaction beneath the adenomatous structures on the surface of the polyp. H.E., x 40

Because of submucosal invasion of the malignant cells, he eventually underwent a partial sigmoidectomy and the resected specimen did not show any evidence of tumor.

Case 13 Polypectomy for pedunculated polyp

A 55-year-old male. *Chief complaint:* bloody stools. He presented with rectal bleeding and later was found to have a pedunculated polyp on barium enema.

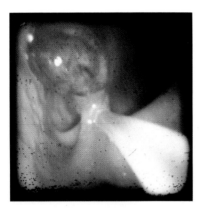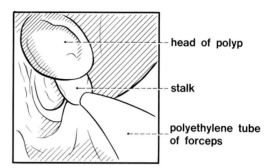

head of polyp

stalk

polyethylene tube of forceps

A. Colonoscopic polypectomy was performed.

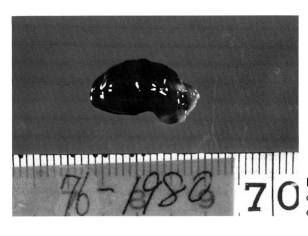

B. The removed specimen shows the body of the polyp on the left and a whitish stalk on the right.

Case 14   Colonic polyposis : familial polyposis

A 39-year-old male. *Chief complaints:* frequent bloody stools and weight loss for the past four months, associated with occasional bloody stools.

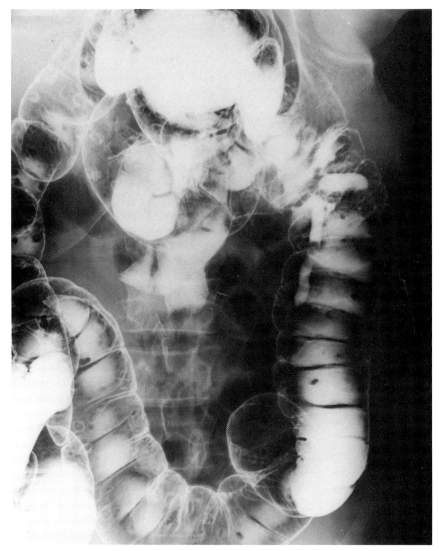

A. Barium enema reveals diffuse polyposis throughout the colon and rectum.

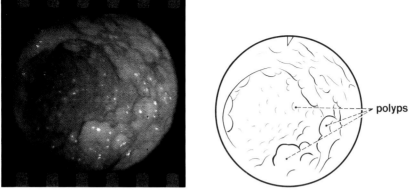

B. Colonoscopy demonstrates numerous polyps, sessile or pedunculated, from the rectum through the 50 cm examined. Biopsy revealed tubular adenoma with moderate atypia in some polyps.

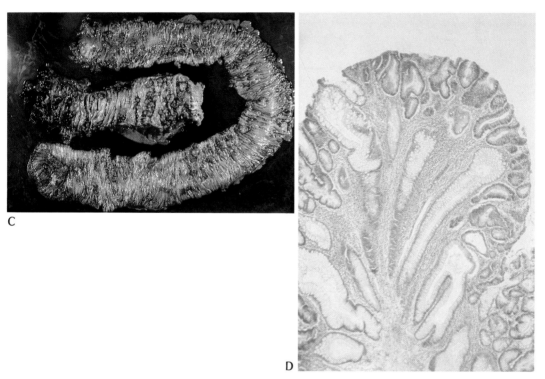

C

D

C. A total proctocolectomy was performed and the resected specimen shows numerous polyps.
D. The histological examination of the polyps reveals carcinoma in adenoma in one rectal polyp, severe atypia in another rectal polyp, and adenoma in the other polyps. H.E., x 40

Case 15   Early colonic carcinoma

A 24-year-old female. *Chief complaint:* mucobloody diarrhea. She developed bloody diarrhea lasting for two weeks. The first barium enema was negative. Sigmoidoscopy revealed a tiny sessile polyp at 20 cm. She again developed rectal bleeding one year later. Sigmoidoscopy at that time again revealed a small polyp without bleeding. Four years later, she developed mucobloody diarrhea.

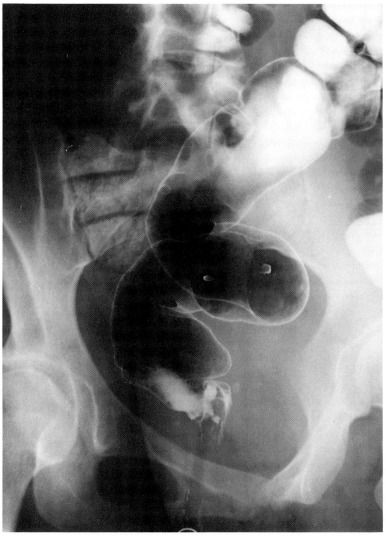

A. Barium enema reveals a sessile polyp in the rectosigmoid.

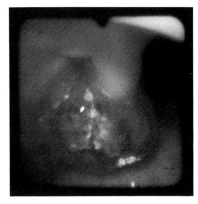 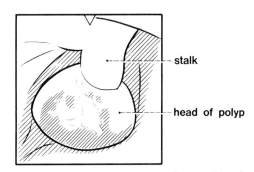

stalk

head of polyp

B. Colonoscopy reveals another larger pedunculated polyp at 40 cm and a smaller sessile polyp at 20 cm noted on barium enema.

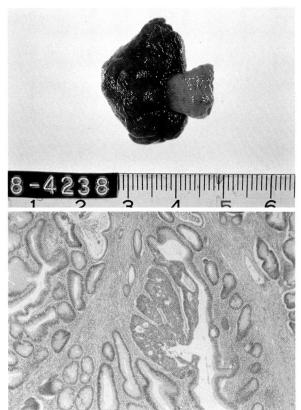

C. The resected specimen obtained by surgical polypectomy.

D. The histological examination demonstrates a focal malignancy confined to the mucosa. H.E., x 100

Case 16   **Polypoid carcinoma**

A 41-year-old male. *Chief complaint:* diarrhea of two months' duration with occasional rectal bleeding.

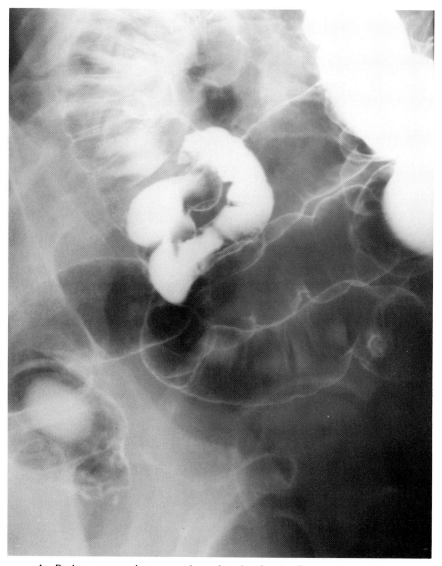

A. Barium enema shows a pedunculated polyp in the sigmoid colon.

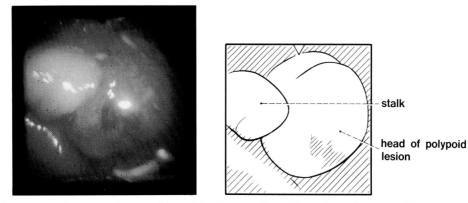

B. Colonoscopy demonstrates a polyp with a long stalk at 78 cm from the anus. The appearance of the tip of the polyp is smooth, most likely suggesting a benign polyp. However, biopsy showed adenocarcinoma from the tip of the polyp.

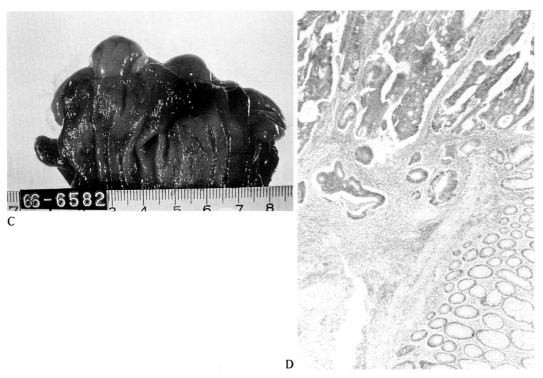

C. Segmental sigmoidectomy was performed and the excised tumor measures 1.0 x 0.8 x 0.5 cm with a 1.5 cm stalk.

D. Histological examination demonstrates a well-differentiated adenocarcinoma with invasion to the submucosal layer. No lymph node involvement is found. H.E., x 40

Case 17   Ulcerated colonic carcinoma

A 51-year-old male. *Chief complaint:* lower abdominal pain of two months' duration.

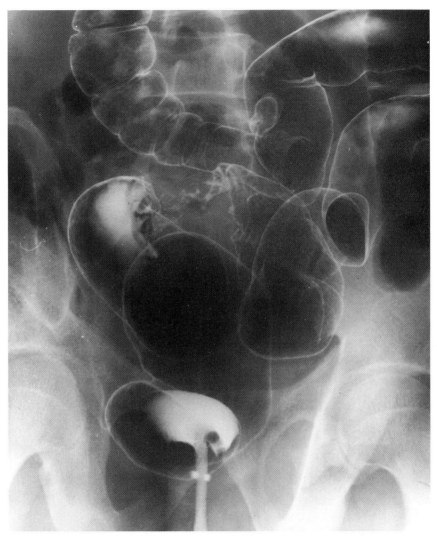

A. Barium enema reveals an applecore lesion in the lower sigmoid colon.

273

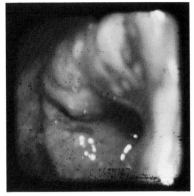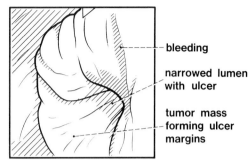

B. Colonoscopy reveals an annular ulcerated mass 20 cm from the anus.

bleeding

narrowed lumen
with ulcer

tumor mass
forming ulcer
margins

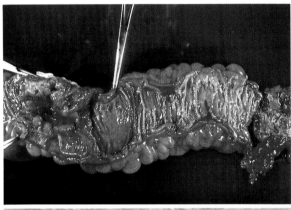

C. The gross specimen of a partial colectomy shows a 6.5 x 5.3 cm ulcerated tumor.

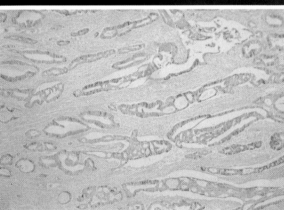

D. The histological examination demonstrates that the tumor is a well-differentiated adenocarcinoma invading the serosa. H.E., x 40

Case 18   **Rectal carcinoid**

A 53-year-old male. *Chief complaint:* bloody stools. He presented with rectal bleeding after defecation. Digital examination of the rectum revealed a sessile polypoid lesion on the right posterior wall 8 cm from the anus.

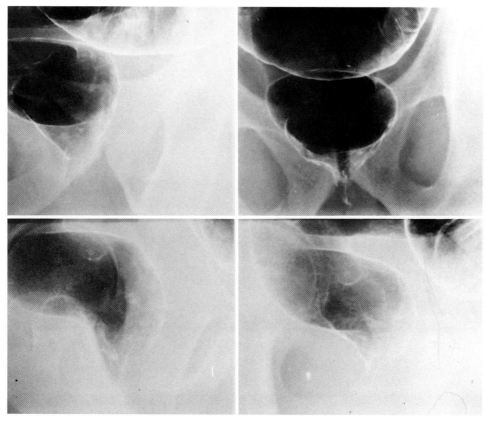

A. Barium enema reveals the presence of a lesion.

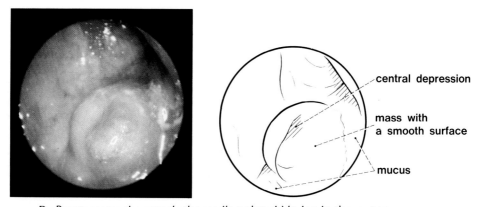

central depression

mass with
a smooth surface

mucus

B. Proctoscopy also reveals the sessile polypoid lesion in the rectum.

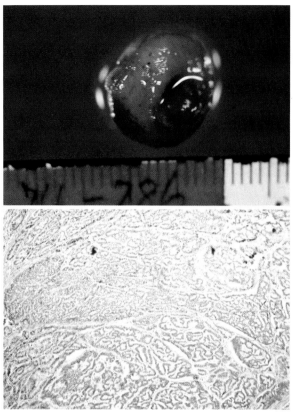

C. Surgical polypectomy through the anus was performed and the polypoid mass removed is sessile with a central depression and 1.2 cm in diameter.

D. Histological study demonstrates a carcinoid tumor which is predominantly trabecular in arrangement, having few areas of the more solid cribriform growth pattern. The nuclei of tumor cells are spherical and evenly basophilic and cytoplasmic margins are indistinct. H.E., x 40

Case 19   Colitis cystica profunda

A 64-year-old female. *Chief complaints:* abdominal pain and constipation for eight months. Three months prior to the first hospital visit, she developed tenesmus followed by a mucobloody stool discharge two months later.

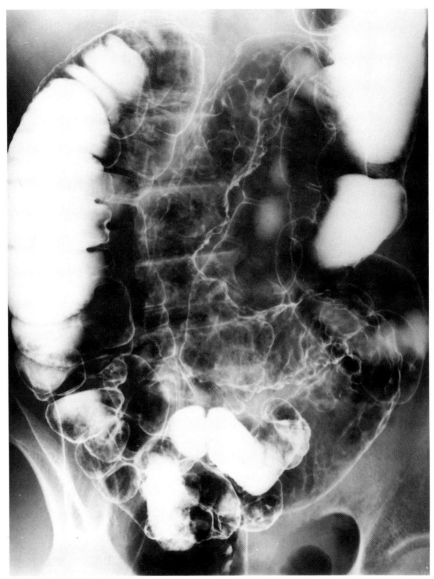

A. Barium enema shows multiple mucosal projections with prominent irregularities of the wall of the rectosigmoid.

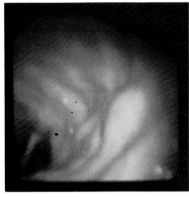 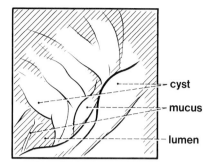

B. Colonoscopy reveals multiple sessile polypoid lesions of varying diameter, distributed from 15 to 50 cm from the anus. The overlying mucosa appears inflamed, tapering smoothly to the surrounding mucosa.

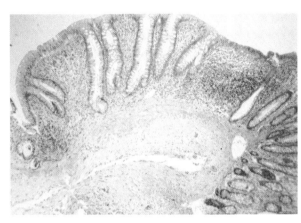

C. Microscopic examination of the biopsy specimen demonstrates some cysts lined by columnar epithelium in the submucosa associated with moderate inflammation in the stroma; the individual lining cells of the cysts are well-differentiated, ruling out the possibility of adenocarcinoma. The most accurate diagnosis is colitis cystica profunda. H.E., x 40

Case 20   Rectal endometriosis

A 37-year-old female. *Chief complaint:* mucobloody stools. Digital examination of the rectum found a protruded mass on the anterior wall 10 cm from the anus which was fixed to the uterus.

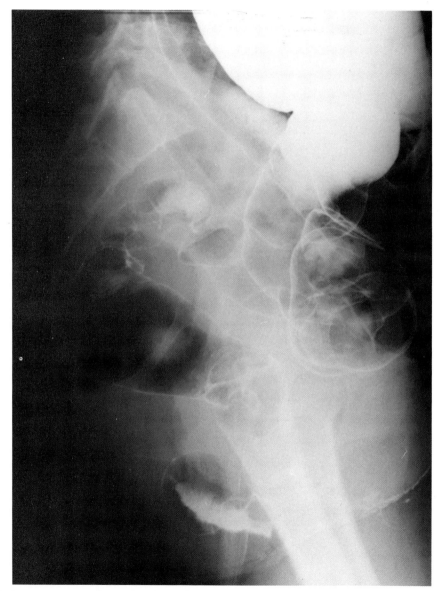

A. Barium enema reveals an anterior wall tumor with a shallow ulceration, 7 cm long, from 10 cm upward. The diagnostic impression is most likely a uterine tumor invading the rectum. However, the possibility of a primary rectal cancer is not ruled out.

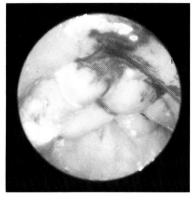 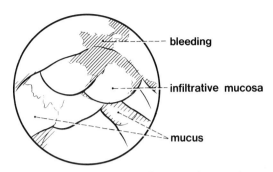

B. Proctoscopic observation reveals a tumor mass of submucosal type, localized on the anterior wall about 11 cm from the anus. A rectal endometriosis was suspected, but a biopsy was negative for endometriosis.

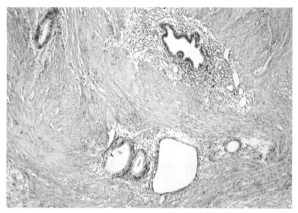

C. The histological examination of the removed uterus proves rectal endometriosis.

Case 21 Colonic diverticulosis

A 75-year-old female. *Chief complaint:* bloody stools. She presented with massive rectal bleeding and subsequently received 8 units of whole blood.

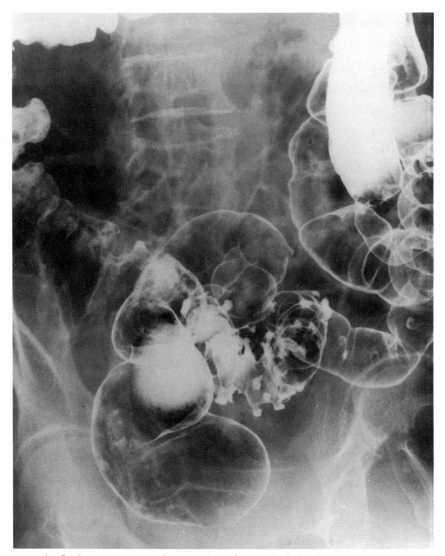

A. Barium enema reveals a number of diverticula in the sigmoid colon.

281

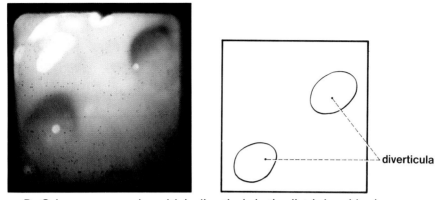

B. Colonoscopy reveals multiple diverticula in the distal sigmoid colon.

Case 22   Rectal carcinoma and colonic diverticula

A 51-year-old female. *Chief complaint:* bloody stools.

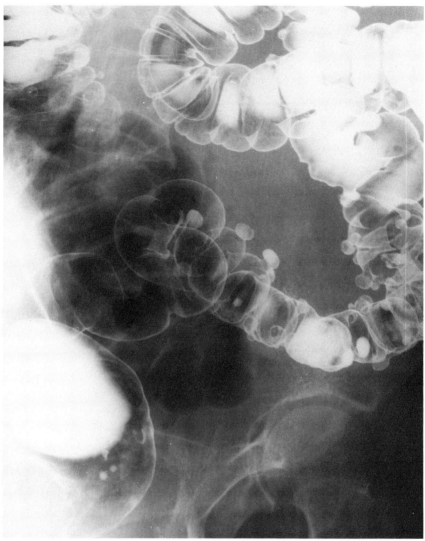

A. Barium enema demonstrates a polypoid tumor of the rectum and diverticulosis of the sigmoid colon.

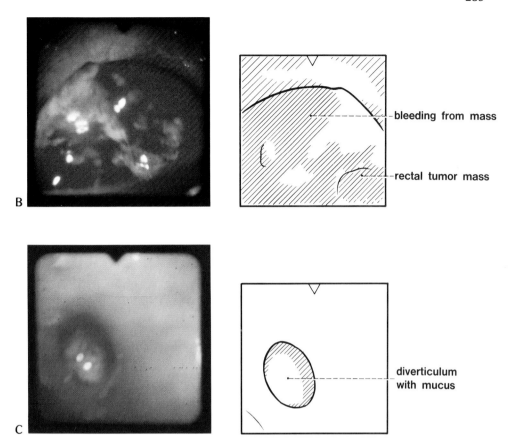

B and C. Colonoscopy reveals a rectal mass on the posterior wall 13 cm from the anus and multiple diverticula proximal to the rectal mass. Biopsy demonstrated adenocarcinoma from the mass.

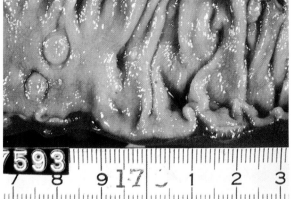

D. Abdominoperineal resection was performed and the resected specimen shows a 2.5 x 2.1 x 1.0 cm rectal mass and multiple diverticula of the sigmoid colon.

Case 23 **Melanosis coli**

A 64-year-old male. *Chief complaint:* long-standing constipation. He is a long-term user of cathartics for more than 20 years. Barium enema was unremarkable.

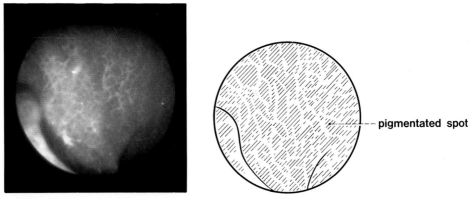

pigmentated spot

A. Colonoscopy reveals a number of dark spots throughout the 40 cm of rectal and sigmoid mucosa examined.

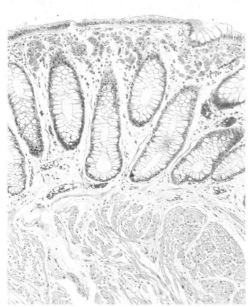

B. Biopsy reveals the presence of phagocytes with pigment in the lamina propria of the rectal mucosa. H.E., x 100

Index

Page numbers in baldface indicate illustrations or tables.